Hospital-based palliative care teams

The hospital-hospice interface

Hospital-based palliative care teams

The hospital-hospice interface

Second Edition

Edited by

R.J. DUNLOP

Medical Director
St Christopher's Hospice, London

and

J.M. HOCKLEY

Clinical Nurse Specialist
Western General Hospital, Edinburgh

OXFORD   NEW YORK   MELBOURNE
OXFORD UNIVERSITY PRESS
1998

Oxford University Press, Great Clarendon Street, Oxford OX2 6DP

Oxford New York

Athens Auckland Bangkok Bogota Bombay Buenos Aires Calcutta
Cape Town Chennai Dar es Salaam Delhi Florence Hong Kong Istanbul
Karachi Kuala Lumpur Madrid Melbourne Mexico City Mumbai
Nairobi Paris São Paolo Singapore Taipei Tokyo Toronto Warsaw
and associated companies in
Berlin Ibadan

Oxford is a registered trade mark of Oxford University Press

Published in the United States
by Oxford University Press Inc., New York

First edition published as Terminal Care Support Teams 1990
Second edition published as Hospital-based Palliative Care Teams: the hospital/hospice interface 1998

A catalogue record for this book is available from the British Library

Library of Congress Cataloging in Publication Data

Hospital-based palliative care teams : the hospital hospice interface
/ edited by R.J. Dunlop and J.M. Hockley.—2nd ed.
Rev. ed. of: Terminal care support teams. 1990.
Includes bibliographical references and index.
1. Terminally ill—Hospital care.   I. Dunlop, R. J. (Robert J.)
II. Hockley, J. M.
[DNLM: 1. Palliative Care.   2. Patient Care Team.   3. Hospital–
Patient Relations.   4. Hospice Care.   WB 310 H8289 1998]
RA1000.H68   1998   362.1'75—dc21   98-22223
ISBN 0 19 262980 8 (Pbk)

Typeset by Joshua Associates Ltd., Oxford
Printed in Great Britain on acid-free paper by
Biddles Ltd, Guildford & King's Lynn

Preface

When the first edition of this book was written (under the name *Terminal care support teams*), there were only a handful of advisory palliative care teams working in hospitals. Since then, the number of teams has grown rapidly. Although the concept of these teams is more widely accepted, there is an even greater need for information about how to set them up, how they work, and how effective they are. The challenges of bringing palliative care into the acute hospital setting have become more complex. The range of diagnostic and treatment options continue to escalate rapidly, throwing up ever more difficult ethical issues. At the same time, financial resources are becoming more limited. The emphasis is on 'value for money' and palliative care has to compete alongside all the other specialties. These issues have lead to a growing demand for this second edition.

We want to apologize for the delay in this edition coming to print. It has been very difficult finding the time to sit down and write while working full-time in palliative care. However, we believe that this practical experience of dealing with day-to-day issues gives this book greater credibility. The theoretical discussions about the dynamics of teamwork, supporting staff at ward level, or working at the cutting edge of end-of-life decision-making are all balanced with practical advice and examples. In addition, we have expanded some important topics. For example, there is a separate chapter on the process of achieving change without power.

Working in the acute hospital setting is very challenging and demanding. The needs of patients, families, and staff are so obvious. Addressing those needs requires skill, patience and dedication. We have found that the rewards are well worth the effort. We hope that this book will encourage and support others who share the vision for this work. Thanks to all those people who have shared their experiences with us and enabled us to produce a more complete book on hospital-based palliative care teams. Special thanks to David Oxenham and Keith Farrer, colleagues on the Palliative Care Team at the Western General Hospital.

London   R.J.D.
Edinburgh   J.M.H.
March 1998

Contents

Contributors to the First Edition

Wendy Burford RGN BTTA Certificate
Clinical Nurse Specialist (Terminal Care)
Brompton Hospital
London SW5

Robert J. Dunlop MB ChB FRACP
Lecturer in the Care of the Dying
Support Care Team
St Bartholomew's Hospital
London EC1A 7BE

James M.G. Foster MB BS FRCA
Consultant Anaesthetist, Pain Clinic
St Bartholomew's Hospital
London EC1A 7BE

Jacquiline Feld MA BA (Hons) Dip Soc. Admin. CQSW
Social Worker
Support Care Team
St Bartholomew's Hospital
London EC1A 7BE

Ann Goldman MA MB FRCP
CLIC Consultant in Paediatric Palliative Care
Department of Haematology and Oncology
Great Ormond Street Hospital for Children NHS Trust
London WC1N 3JH

Tom Kerrance RGN BTA NAHC
Chief Nursing Officer to
National Heart and Chest Hospital
Brompton Hospital
London SW5

Jo Hockley RGN SCM MSc
Clinical Nurse Specialist (Palliative Care)
Support Care Team
St Bartholomew's Hospital
London EC1A 7BE

Rosemary Lennard MB ChB PhD MRCP
Support Team
St Thomas' Hospital
Lambeth Palace Road
London EC1 7E

Judith Reddy RGN Dip HV
Clinical Nurse Specialist (Palliative Care)
Support Care Team
St Bartholomew's Hospital
London EC1A 7BE

Dame Cicely Saunders OM DBE FRCP
Chairman and Founder
St Christopher's Hospice
Lawrie Park Road
London
SE26 6D2

1

The need for palliative care teams

The writing of this second edition has come from a continuing desire to promote greater understanding of how hospital-based palliative care teams can improve the care of terminally ill patients and their families within the acute setting. Although the first edition was written as a response to setting up one of the 'first-wave' palliative care teams at St Bartholomew's Hospital, London, there is now considerably more experience. Both the literature and personal experience have facilitated a greater awareness of the joys and the sorrows of working in palliative care teams. The most exciting aspect has been to see the greater committment of health professionals as they have become more interested in the challenges presented by patients with incurable diseases and their readiness to be involved.

Palliative care teams would not be where they are now had it not been for the therapies and insights developed within the modern hospice setting. Those involved in the hospice movement of the 1960s would give credit to those who advocated the care of the dying before them. Caring for the dying is nothing new but is constantly evolving. New treatments and new concepts of care are being developed which are relevant to current practice. This book does not contain details about specific treatments, since these have been published already (see Appendix). Rather, this book is about taking and adapting the philosophy of care developed within hospice units and applying it to the hospital environment.

Over the past few years several different names have been given to the evolving concept of a consultancy team advising on the care of dying patients within the acute hospital setting: terminal care support team, symptom control team, support care team, palliative care team. (The word palliative comes from the Latin *palliare*, meaning to cloak.) It would seem that the term **palliative care team** is now used by the majority of hospital-based services. For the sake of convenience, we will use this term throughout the rest of the book. Many such teams also provide a service for terminally ill patients in the community. Although some guidelines in this book are appropriate for home care, we have recommended specialist books on this subject in the Appendix.

The World Health Organization (WHO 1990) drew up a definition of palliative care, stating its goals as follows:

Palliative care is the active total care of patients whose disease is not responsive to curative treatment. Control of pain, of other symptoms, and of psychological, social and spiritual problems is paramount. The goal of palliative care is achievement of the best possbile quality of life for patients an their families. Many aspects of palliative care are also applicable earlier in the course of the illness, in conjunction with anti-cancer treatment. Palliative care:
• affirms life and regards dying as a normal process
• neither hastens nor postpones death
• provides relief from pain and other distressing symptoms
• integrates the psychological and spiritual aspects of patient care
• offers a support system to help patients live as actively as possible until death
• offers a support system to help the family cope during the patient's illness in their own bereavement.

We have chosen to focus on peripatetic hospital-based palliative care teams because they seek to upgrade terminal care without assuming control of patients. This means that palliative care teams can only advise the various medical, surgical, and oncology teams. Bringing the principles of hospice care alongside the disease-oriented hospital system is fraught with difficulties and frustrations. We have drawn upon the experience of several palliative care teams to provide guidelines about coping with and overcoming these difficulties.

Palliative care units (Hoskin and Hanks 1988) can also effect changes in the management of hospital in-patients. They provide a hospice-like setting within the hospital, and frequently offer an advisory service. This book provides some information about palliative care units.

By way of introduction, the next section of this chapter briefly examines the history of terminal care in hospital. The rest of the chapter reviews the needs of dying patients, their families, and professional carers in the acute setting. These needs are the reason why palliative care teams were developed.

How the care of the dying became neglected

In many ways, the history of St Bartholomew's Hospital, London (Barts) provides a good illustration of the change in attitudes towards the care of the dying over the centuries. When Barts was founded in 1123 there was no difference in the meaning of 'hospital' and 'hospice'. The original Hospital house was a large hall in close proximity to the chapel. Rest and shelter were provided for the sick poor of London. The depth of commitment to the patients was evidenced by the Master of the Priory visiting them daily. As with many modern hospices, volunteers played an important role in the care of patients, and there was considerable reliance on charitable donations of money and food.

It is interesting to note that even at this time, the Hospital was associated with the possibility of cure. Early case studies document the resolution of a woman's swollen tongue when Rahere, the founder of Barts, placed a relic of the Cross upon it. The Book of the Foundation reports how 'some man joyed with jubilation at the remedy of his aching head, another for reparation of his going that he lacked'. The recognition of this potential for healing was not confined to the medical fraternity. Even in the twelfth century, seriously ill people would undertake arduous journeys from all over England in the hope of a cure. The determination of some patients to pursue even the slimmest hope is still very evident today.

After 400 years as a monastic hospital Barts was re-established on a secular basis and granted a new charter by King Henry VIII. In 1539 Thomas Vicary, a surgeon, described the palliative function of Barts to King Henry VIII. The Hospital was 'for the ayde and comforte of the poore, sykke, blynde, aged, and impotent persones beying not hable to helpe themselffs nor havying any place certeyn whereyn they may be lodged, cherysshed, or refresshed', to which he added 'tyll they be cured and holpen of theyre dyseases and syknesse' (Moore 1918).

It is frequently held nowadays that technological advances have prejudiced the care of the dying. However, attitudes of medical attendants appeared to have changed as early as 1544. The Royal Charter outlined the duties of the various staff involved in the care of patients at Barts. The role of the surgeons was 'to see if the patient were curable or not, so that none should be admitted who were incurable, none rejected who were curable' (Moore 1918). During the time of the Great Plague, physicians and surgeons distanced themselves by moving to the safety of the countryside. The care of patients was abandoned to 'the matron and apothecary' (Hector 1974).

Although the change in attitudes towards the incurable predated the greatest explosion of medical science and technology which began in the early part of this century, there has been an increasingly optimistic climate about trying further treatments for the very sick. As a direct result, one of the outcomes over the last 70 years has been the greater number of patients gravitating towards hospital care. This has resulted in more people being cared for in hospital. There has also been a dramatic shift to more people dying in hospital rather than in their own homes. Swings of the pendulum tend to be redressed by society at large and it would seem no coincidence that the new hospice movment was established at a time when the care of the dying appeared to be neglected at the expense of futile but increasingly burdensome attempts at cure.

The modern hospice movement

Although Mme Jeanne Garnier opened the first hospice, especially for the dying, in France during the middle of the nineteenth century, it was not until the 1890s that Dr Howard Barrett, founder of St Luke's Home for the Dying Poor, tried to reach the public's interest in England (Saunders 1988) and steps were first taken to redress the imbalance. The Irish Sisters of Charity, having founded their first hospice in Dublin, established St Joseph's Hospice in close proximity to Barts Hospital, and the first in-patient was accepted in 1905. Since then, St Joseph's has continually had to expand and it now has over 60 beds for specialist palliative care. Physical, psychological, and spiritual support became key elements of a theme of total care for terminally ill patients and their families.

Hospice care took on a new dimension with the opening of St Christopher's Hospice in 1966. The restoration of the caring art of medicine was coupled with the sensitive application of the scientific method. In addition, there was a commitment to teaching the newfound knowledge and expertise. The number of hospices has increased rapidly since then, both nationally and internationally. The contribution of the hospice movement to current medical practice cannot be doubted.

As hospice practice developed in the UK, many patients admitted to hospice with distressing pain and other symptoms were able to be discharged back to their own home. This precipitated the need for hospices to develop their own home care teams. Specialist nurses visited patients in their own homes, advising general practitioners and district nurses about the care of the dying. This ripple effect out into the community spread throughout the country. Then, at the end of the 1970s, palliative care started to come full circle back into acute care with the formation of hospice teams within the hospital (see Fig. 1.1).

In 1976 St Thomas's Hospital, London formed the first hospital-based

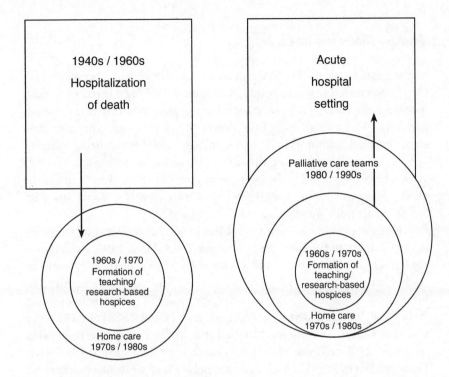

Fig. 1.1. Evolution of palliative care.

terminal care support team in the UK (Bates *et al.* 1981). It was based on a model from St Luke's Hospital, New York (Kaplan and O'Connor 1989). The development of a palliative care team at Barts represented a seed of the modern hospice movement in the oldest medieval hospital in the U.K. The balance is being adjusted to incorporate the terminally ill once again.

It was important for hospices to stand outside the established National Health Service hospital structure in the UK before being recognized for the care they were able to offer. Dame Cicely Saunders (1993) acknowledged that 'The first modern [hospice] units . . . saw themselves as examples of ways of giving appropriate care rather than as models to be copied . . . a major aim was to define principles that could be interpreted according to various settings'. Now, 30 years on, it is exciting to see hospice care come full circle as it establishes itself within the acute hospital in the form of peripatetic hospital-based palliative care teams.

Terminal illness and hospitals

The importance of the hospice movement has caused some people to lose their perspective on where people die. It must be remembered that most hospice units hardly take any patients dying from non-malignant disease and only 14% of those dying from cancer. It has been our experience that some hospital administrators and clinicians point to existing hospice services to avoid confronting the care of the dying in hospital. There will always be people dying in the acute setting of a hospital. To try and place all the dying in hospice units, even if this were possible, would again be hiding death from society.

Where people die has been the subject of several studies (Cartwright *et al.* 1973, Lunt and Hillier 1981, Bowling 1983, Herd 1990, Addington-Hall *et al.* 1991, Axelsson and Christensen 1996). In their nationwide study Cartwright *et al.* (1973) found that 52% of *all* deaths occurred in hospitals or institutions. Since then the percentage of cancer patients dying in hospital has increased to 60% (Lunt and Hillier 1981). In 1987 the Office of Census and Surveys detailed that 56% of deaths were in NHS hospitals, 27% at home and 17% 'elsewhere' which included hospices. Field and James (1993) concluded that only 4% of all deaths (cancer and non-cancer) occurred in hospice units. There is some variation between urban and semi-rural areas but there is still a large majority of deaths occurring in institutions.

Patients with cancer, stroke, respiratory disease, and uncommon illnesses will tend to die in hospital (Bowling 1983). Up to 40% of hospital deaths are related to ischaemic heart disease (Wilkes 1984). Cancer accounts for one third of hospital deaths. The majority of discharged patients are followed up by out-patient clinics, with at least half being seen on more than one occasion (Cartwright *et al.* 1973).

It would appear that most professionals, as well as patients and families, often want a death to occur at home, but considerable expertise and support are required to enable this to happen. Poorly controlled pain and other symptoms, and exhaustion of the lay carer, are the two main reasons for terminally ill cancer patients being admitted from home to hospital (Herd 1990). Over 80% of out-patients have symptoms that cause relatives considerable concern. Admission can also be influenced by duration and nature of illness, lack of medical help/support and accessible emergency help, fear of sole responsibility, and fear of the unexpected (Bowling 1983). In a more recent study by Cartwright (1991), hospital consultants and community nurses wanted more people to die at home but general practitioners were not so sure.

Patients who are unmarried, who are wives rather than husbands, who have been ill for between three months and two years rather than two years or more, who are under 45 years of age, and who are without children are most likely to die in hospital (Cartwright *et al.* 1973, Bowling and Cartwright 1982). Many terminally ill patients have a relatively short stay in hospital. One third of patients will die within a week of final admission. However, 40% will be in hospital for longer than a month (Wilkes 1984). This is considerably longer than the average length of stay for other patients in acute beds. Doctors often become concerned that dying patients 'block' the use of these beds and will want these patients discharged or transferred.

Terminally ill patients are less likely to die in teaching hospitals because the discharge rate is higher. Patients who die in teaching hospitals tend to be younger, 50% being under the age of 65, compared with 30% in district general hospitals (Cartwright *et al.* 1973). This is because younger patients are less likely to passively accept a terminal illness and will seek active treatment at a teaching hospital.

There appear to be a number of reasons that have promoted the establishment of hospital-based palliative care teams.

- Despite the establishment of hospices and home care teams, most people still die in hospital.
- The unpredictability of the terminal phase of non-malignant diseases means that admission to hospital is likely in case the patient's deterioration is not a terminal event; unless patients and their families have had the opportunity to understand the advanced nature of the disease and end-of-life decisions have been raised.
- Patients with a non-malignant disease are unlikely to be accommodated within a hospice setting precisely because of the unpredictable prognosis.
- Hospice education needs to be given where the majority of people die, because that is where care professionals are exposed to the issues in their training. Too often the people attending hospice education are those nurses, doctors, social workers who are already converts to the practice of palliative care. Hospice education needs to go out to meet those caring for the dying as part of their day-to-day surgical/medical practice. The peripatetic hospital-based palliative care team therefore not only plays an important part in advising good palliation of symptoms while patients remain in the acute setting but should also be part of the education of nurses and doctors while in training.

Why do patients die in hospital?

Whether administrators like it or not, the majority of patients are still dying in the acute hospital setting. It is our opinion that until there are better services for the dying patient and family with access to specialist palliative care advice, both within the acute hospital setting as well as in the community, this will continue to happen. Not enough is done within most hospital settings to expedite the necessary care and advice for dying patients and their families.

Mount *et al.* (1974) found that health professionals, including nurses and social workers, felt that it was inappropriate for terminally ill patients to occupy acute hospital beds. The only group in favour were the terminally ill patients themselves. Many people start with the premise that patients prefer to die at home because of the familiar surroundings. One reason patients favour being in hospital is the sense of security, especially if symptoms are not properly controlled (Herd 1990). Wilkes (1984) found relatives shared this view and felt hospital provided better care. However, a more recent prospective study by Townsend *et al.* (1990) found that 58% of cancer patients at first interview wanted to die at home. This figure decreased to 49% as the illness progressed and death was imminent. The final outcome showed that 29% of patients died at home with 57% dying in hospital. All patients were selected from within an area well served by both hospice and home care services.

Bowling (1983) states that patients need to be fully informed about their illness in order to choose where they want to die. She felt that often the patient was the last person to be informed, if at all. Interestingly, Townsend *et al.* reported that 90% of patients were aware of their diagnosis and at least 95% of these knew their long term if not their immediate prognosis. Why is it, therefore, that patients still die in hospital? Any specialist palliative care team working in the acute setting wants to be able to fulfil the wishes of those under their care, especially if it relates to where they would like to die. Yes, there may be difficulties getting resources in the community alerted quickly, especially if the lay carer is elderly, but is this the only reason?

We undertook a prospective study of 100 patients to determine why, despite being under our care, these patients still died in hospital (Dunlop *et al.* 1989). The reason why a patient died in hospital was determined by the team member who had been most involved in the care. Patients had been referred to the specialist palliative care team for advice primarily concerning symptom control issues.

Thirty-three patients died while receiving treatments such as radio-therapy and chemotherapy, or were being investigated for first presentation of advanced disease. Their deterioration was relatively unexpected. It might be thought that these patients were subjected to unnecessary interventions. However, several patients had wanted to continue treatment when the doctors wanted to withdraw. These patients often asked us to convey their feelings to the doctors.

Twenty-four patients wanted to die at home, or in some alternative to hospital. Although plans were set in motion to fulfil their desire, these patients deteriorated too quickly and were unable to travel. A significant number of patients, twenty eight in total, died in hospital because their relatives were unable to cope at home. There were three main reasons why this occurred:

- The patient and relatives denied the illness and made no contingency plans before a crisis of symptoms precipitated admission. These patients and their families were often referred to the palliative care team because their denial was considered 'inappropriate'.
- Some patients were aware of the fact that the relatives were physically or emotionally unable to continue home care. These patients specifically requested admission to hospital. Often a close relationship between patient, family, and ward staff had built up over several admissions.
- Several patients did not specifically choose to die in hospital but refused to consider being transferred elsewhere. The ability to strike up new relationships and adapt to new environments steadily declines as an illness progresses.

Twelve patients were semi-conscious or comatose when referred and were too ill to be transferred elsewhere. Two patients died suddenly of cardiac arrest. One patient wanted to return home but had premonitory carotid artery bleeding so was advised by her doctors against discharge.

It must be stated that the sample clearly was not representative of the wider general hospital experience, because patients were referred in a major teaching hospital. The university hospital setting produces a bias towards a younger patient population reflected in the fact that the average age of our patients at death is at least 8–10 years less than the national average. However, the findings are representative of the work within a university hospital/cancer centre and for that reason are important.

Having said that the majority of patients die in hospital, what are their needs within this setting; what can a palliative care team therefore expect to face?

The needs of patients

Over the last 15 years there have been a few retrospective studies of the needs and care given to people who have died in hospital (Wilkes 1984, Addington-Hall 1991). Houts *et al.* (1988) carried out a prospective study to look at the needs of terminally ill cancer patients at home but studies highlighting the needs of the terminally ill within the acute hospital setting are more scarce.

Symptom control

Two prospective studies have looked at the symptoms of hospital patients with malignant and non-malignant conditions (Hinton 1963; Hockley *et al.* 1988). Both studies revealed that the majority of patients had distressing symptoms.

Many patients had multiple symptoms. The relative frequency of symptoms such as anorexia, pain, breathlessness, and weakness are little different from hospice experience (see Table 1.1). However, sleeplessness was more of a problem because of ward noise and routine turning.

Table 1.1 Symptom profile patients presenting to a palliative care unit (Bruera 1993) versus hospital in-patients prospective study (Hockley *et al.*, 1988)

Symptom	Bruera and Fainsinger[c] (*n* = 275)	Hockley *et al.*[a] (*n* = 26)
	Incidence (%)	
Weakness/fatigue	90	88
Anorexia	85	92
Pain	76	69
Nausea	68	54
Constipation	65	54
Sedation/confusion	60	34
Dyspnoea	12	69[a]
Insomnia		88
Sore mouth		81
Pressure sores		61[b]

[a] Patients all referred from Respiratory Directorate (cancer and non-malignant disease).
[b] Worse in patients with non-malignancies.
[c] Cancer patients only.

Patients with non-malignant disease are just as likely to experience distressing symptoms, in particular anorexia and pressure sores. These patients, however, are less likely to have their symptoms relieved. Symptoms are poorly managed for several reasons:

- patients frequently accept symptoms as inevitable and do not complain
- professionals fail to appreciate the symptoms, particularly the less obvious ones such as nausea, pain, pressure sores and insomnia
- responses to symptoms are often inadequate, e.g. inattention to pressure areas and mouth care
- inadequate and infrequent doses of analgesics and laxatives are prescribed.

Brescia *et al.* (1990) found that 77% of 1103 patients referred to the palliative care team at the Calvary Hospital, New York between July 1985 and June 1986, complained of pain, which was severe in 38% of patients. These results were very similar to data collected by Simpson (1991). She carried out a small research project to facilitate the creation of a hospital-based palliative care team. Over a 6 week period in hospital she interviewed 78 terminally ill patients: 71% of patients complained of pain, which was severe in 36%, and kept 28% of patients awake at night. Out of all the patients she interviewed 69% had uncontrolled symptoms. The worst symptoms were pain, vomiting and anorexia. Sixty nine per cent of patients had difficulty sleeping at night (40% caused by pain, 25% by 'worry', 22% by disturbances through ward routine)

Psychological and spiritual needs

It is well known that multiple distressing physical symptoms will lower pain threshold and mood. Hockley *et al.* (1988) found that the six patients who felt extremely depressed all had high scores on their distressing symptom scale. Hinton (1963) found that at least 50% of terminally ill patients in hospital described themselves as feeling depressed, again particularly patients experiencing a number of distressing symptoms or who were aware that they were dying. At least 75% of patients dying in hospital will indicate to an observer that they are aware of impending death (Hinton 1963); 50% will have talked to their relatives about dying (Hockley *et al.* 1988).

Anxiety was found to be common, particularly in patients who did not know their diagnosis or what was going to happen to them (Hockley 1988). As long ago as the early 1950s, Kelly and Friesen (1950) showed that 89% of cancer patients wanted to be told if the condition was irreversible. Despite this evidence, 88% of doctors in a teaching hospital in the US had a personal policy of not telling (Oken 1961). The doctors allowed their own fears about a potentially fatal illness to determine what they told patients. Mount *et al.* (1974) found that 80% of patients thought they should always 'be told the nature of their disease'. At least two thirds of patients wanted to know the absolute truth about their prognosis.

Anxiety was also associated with some symptoms, particularly breath-lessness. There was an association between anxiety and a tepid religious faith or dependent children. Other important causes of patient stress include the complex technology for treatment and diagnosis, and the prolonged periods of waiting for results of treatments or investigations (Degner and Beaton 1987).

Patients in hospital are more likely to experience anxiety and irritability than patients in hospice (Hinton 1979). At least 25% of patients identify spiritual support as playing a major role in coping with their illness. However, up to 45% of patients say that they are very unlikely to use a service providing spiritual guidance and support (Rainey *et al.* 1980).

Some patients do not have relatives or carers to help them. This can add to their distress and loneliness. The proportion of patients who have no relatives or carers is approximately 20–27% (Addington-Hall *et al.* 1991). For patients with a relatively short prognosis who have no close carers, the hospice is the ideal place of care if the patient is willing to go.

The next section reviews relatives' needs, some of which are specific to the hospital setting.

The needs of relatives

Physical symptoms

Hockley *et al.* (1988) found that fatigue was the most common symptom experienced by relatives. In addition, up to 20% of relatives developed a physical illness because of the stress of coping. Within the hospital setting this aspect of caring for relatives is often ignored. Relatives therefore come to the hospital sometimes twice a day to be with their loved one. It is not surprising that they feel physically tired and often find it harder to cope emotionally.

Psychological needs

Depression and anxiety result from the threatened loss of the patient. This stress is heightened when patients say they are probably going to die. Hockley *et al.* (1988) reported that 50% of relatives reported that their loved one had openly talked about dying with them but they had not told anyone. Relatives are often not prepared for this and find themselves changing the subject or trying to be optimistic, only to subsequently feel depressed because of the breakdown in a trusting relationship.

Lack of information makes these emotions worse. Relatives receive conflicting statements about the patient's condition and prognosis (Hockley *et al.* 1988). Relatives may be desperate for more information but do not make this desire known. They are afraid to disrupt the busy routine of the doctors and nurses. Poor communication also results from the lack of continuity of care by ward staff and the frequent changes in junior medical staff.

We found that many relatives fear the patient will be discharged home (Hockley *et al.* 1988). This fear was related to the patient's distressing symptoms and the perceived lack of general practitioner support. Relatives were also afraid of the patient falling or dying at home. At the same time, relatives felt guilty because they were not able to look after the patient at home. They saw this as letting the patient down. There is much that members of a palliative care team can do to calm these fears:

- organizing a family meeting with members of the ward team
- asking junior medical staff to speak to the general practitioner
- speaking directly to the district nurse and/or hospice nurse/Macmillan nurse after the ward have informed them of the discharge
- helping ward staff to make proper discharge plans on appropriate days of the week.

Dissatisfaction with hospital care during the final illness was reported by 50% of relatives (Addington-Hall *et al.* 1991). Disappointment arose over two main issues, firstly the lack of nurses to provide adequate care and inadequate pain control. Thirty seven per cent of relatives also felt dissatisfied with insufficient information by hospital personnel and the way it was given. Carers had wanted more information about the patient's condition and felt that they had not been warned that death was imminent.

In the case of more elderly relatives, Bowling (1983) found that 59% of the surviving bereaved people who were not present at the deaths of their spouses were upset at being absent. They had wanted to say goodbye. One person had been at the hospital for eight or nine days without leaving the bedside: it was then suggested she go home for a couple of hours, during which time the husband died. The experience of nursing staff in recognizing the imminence of death is so important.

Anger is often deflected away from the immediate situation on to social problems such as difficulties in transport and noisy neighbours. After the patient dies, up to 20% of relatives will criticize the hospital as being uncaring (Wilkes 1984). It is less common for relatives to lodge a written complaint. Even so, complaints about the care of dying patients had consituted 8% of the total number of complaints received by Barts' administration before the setting up of the palliative care team.

Relatives' distress may be increased by the routine hospital procedures after a death. A requests for a postmortem examination may be accompanied by veiled threats of a coroner's enquiry if the family do not agree. Being given new information when one is shocked and numb after the death of a loved one is often difficult to remember. For a palliative care team/nurse specialist just starting within a hospital the drawing up of a 'bereavement booklet' (see chapter 6) can be extremely useful. Staff have even been asked to help redesign the 'viewing chapel'.

Many relatives find the task of picking up the patient's belongings in a property bag or patient's clothing bag very upsetting. Some hospitals have now produced more appropriate plain bags.

These problems all contribute to the impact of bereavement. Wright *et al.* (1988) have written an excellent review about the difficulties of the bereaved in hospital.

Social needs

Many progressive debilitating illnesses will have profound effects on the structure and integrity of the patient and family. Often there is no longer the extended family to help because people have moved away to seek jobs and careers. Besides not having close family around, younger patients may lose earning power, with important financial consequences.

Marital and family relationships may well come under strain because of the redistribution of roles, and changes in the patient's sexuality. Social isolation, precipitated by the decline in strength and motivation of the patient, will compound these disruptive effects.

It is important that members of the palliative care team are aware of the needs of ethnic minorities. Often nurses and doctors on the ward are ignorant about different cultural needs of the dying Hindu, Sikh, or Muslim patient and family (Firth 1993). Team members can pass on knowledge and be involved in translating the needs of these patients within the busy ward environment. This can enable ward staff take more time to understand the different cultural needs.

Bereavement can be very isolating unless close friends and family are around to encourage and help. Adjusting to loss is difficult enough but made worse if there have been problems within the acute hospital setting that have caused anger or disappointment to the bereaved. When a patient has spent many weeks in a hospital there is a danger that the relative will become isolated from the community. The risk of further isolation may precipitate the need for bereavement support.

The needs of professional carers

Hospital staff are affected by patients' and relatives' problems. Being aware of staff needs is essential for a balanced approach to the care of the dying in hospital. Good palliative care at the ward level depends on well-informed and well-supported staff.

Nurses

Nursing staff are the professional carers who have closest contact with terminally ill patients and their families. Forty per cent of student nurses find caring for the dying stressful; the remainder consider it 'rewarding but stressful at times' (Hockley 1989). Distressing physical symptoms, particularly pain and breathlessness, are very alarming for junior nurses. If nurses lack knowledge about treatments or pain/symptom control, they will try to avoid dying patients. Procedures such as dressing fungating wounds or dealing with incontinence are not usually considered stressful, unless there is insufficient time to perform them.

Many junior nurses find the psychological care of the dying difficult. This may also lead them to withdraw from the dying. Often wards are very busy, and spending time explaining to and/or comforting an anxious patient can increase stress if there are other jobs that need to be done. The stress will increase when a nurse is not confident she is reassuring appropriately. The patient who asks difficult questions about diagnosis and dying can often catch nurses 'off guard', forcing them to give an inadequate answer, which in turn makes the nurse feel disappointed.

Anxiety is the commonest emotional response to stress. First-year nurses tend to be anxious about the difficulty of controlling their own emotions. More experienced students and trained staff are anxious about their responsibility toward the patient and relative. Depression and anger may occur, and nurses will sometimes feel 'overwhelmed'. It is rare, however, for these feelings to make nurses want to give up nursing or go 'off sick' (Hockley 1989).

Nurses often lack support from other staff, including other nurses, supervisors, and doctors. When doctors find it difficult to make or communicate decisions about the management of patients, nurses bear the brunt of relatives' questions and anger. Disagreements about treatment decisions may also exacerbate stress, particularly when aggressive treatments are continued into the terminal phase and are seen as unwarranted (Degner and Beaton 1987). The converse may also apply, for example when patients' symptoms are ignored, or when potential treatments are denied patients who are still relatively well. This may not be so much of a problem with nurses working in hospices, but it is clearly more of an issue within the acute hospital setting.

Nurses frequently emphasize the need for more teaching about the care of the dying. First- and second-year student nurses want to learn how to cope with their own feelings and reactions. They also want to learn how to talk to dying patients, not just to answer difficult questions but to facilitate ordinary conversation, while performing a bed bath for example. Senior student nurses want to learn about how to deal with families, especially when a patient has died (Hockley 1989). Qualified nurses realize that they can influence treatment decisions and want more details about symptom control.

Doctors

Maguire (1985) discusses how psychological care can be blocked by health care professionals, own attitudes, vulnerabilities, and fears. This results in distancing tactics and avoidance. One study showed that surgeons spend less time at the foot of beds of patients whose surgery has been unsuccessful (Knight and Field 1981). Doctors find it very stressful making decisions about continuing or stopping treatment of patients who are likely to die (Degner and Beaton 1987). They often do not feel confident to ask patients how they see the situation themselves. Being more open with the patient can help to clarify the next step in care. Stress is increased by the feeling that other doctors are waiting to point out mistakes which might have contributed to the patient's decline. Doctors seldom discuss these feelings with each other. If doctors are less paternalistic, able to discuss more with dying patients and their families, and become more confident in end-of-life decision-making (see chapter 5), patients and families will become more familiar with making choices about further treatment and place of care.

Lack of knowledge about symptom control also contributes to a sense of helplessness in medical staff. This results in terminally ill patients being ignored during ward rounds. It is little wonder that symptoms are under-detected, and that doctors over-report anxiety as a problem for patients (Wilkes 1984). By default, junior doctors often have to assume the care of these patients. Yet, up to 50% of junior doctors report that they have received inadequate training to enable them to cope with the care of the dying (Ahmedzai 1982). Junior staff find themselves having to act as go-between for ward nurses and consultants. The stress of having to report unwelcome problems to their seniors may be considerable.

Many experience anger and frustration when patients deteriorate despite treatment. In the past doctors have often coped with death by avoiding patients once they have begun to die. Despite increasing opportunity to learn about aspects of symptom control and communicating with dying patients, often only professionals who already have an interest and grasp of caring for the dying attend such lectures. More education and support must be given to doctors within the acute hospital setting as part of their continuing training.

Other carers

Staff from a wide range of disciplines have a valuable role to play in the care of the dying (NAHA 1987). Physiotherapists, occupational therapists, social workers, chaplains, dieticians, psychologists, and psychiatrists should be involved as necessary. Weekly multidisciplinary ward meetings or ward rounds can be a very useful way of discussing the needs of dying patients and the particular role for the wider multidisciplinary team. After a death has occurred on the ward it is important to notify those of the wider team that have been involved. These staff may have contributed a lot, both emotionally and professionally, to the care of the patient. Too often that contribution is forgotten and they are just left to find out details at a later date. This undermines morale and prevents other staff from feeling part of a valued team.

Translating needs into team objectives

It is important to stress that every health professional should have the necessary core skills to care for the dying. Finley and Jones (1995) has identified three levels of intervention:the palliative approach, palliative interventions, and specialist palliative care.

- The palliative approach is relevant to all patients and their families with incurable conditions. The emphasis is on holistic care, which should be a core skill of every health professional.
- A palliative intervention is used to maintain a good quality of life. It is a non-curative treatment aimed at improving symptoms. Examples include palliative surgery such as the formation of a colostomy, or palliative radiotherapy for the treatment of bone metastases. The intervention is monitored by the specialists performing the intervention.
- Specialist palliative care is delivered by clinicians with specialist palliative care training. It is multidisciplinary and forms the basis of care given by those working in hospice, home care teams, Macmillan nurses and hospital-based palliative care teams.

At the hospital or ward level, there should be a philosophy and objectives of care for dying patients and their families. This committment should underpin a hospital-based palliative care team's objectives. It is important that the hospital acknowledges the role of a palliative care team and supports the changes needed to fulfil this role. If not, any team objectives will soon be frustrated.

An example of a hospital's philosophy and objectives of palliative care is:

The aim throughout the . . . NHS Trust is to provide effective palliative care to patients and their families by:
- removing or alleviating unpleasant symptoms and suffering
- addressing the fear and isolation of patients who are faced with a life-threatening illness
- maintaining quality of life, to enable the person to live as normal as life as possible for as long as possible
- involving the chaplaincy department and spiritual advisors in recognizing the spiritual needs of patients and their families
- involving patients and families in making choices about their future care
- ensuring continuity of care and promoting a seamless service with community services and specialist palliative care units
- ensuring privacy when death occurs

- providing the necessary support and information to the family
- recognizing the need for open and honest communication with the patient and family at all times
- providing a high standard of palliative care through a multidisciplinary team approach
- involving specialist expertise through the hospital-based palliative care team when necessary.

No specialist palliative care team can work without its own clear objectives. The needs found in the hospital provide the basis for the aims of any palliative care team:

- To work alongside the ward team caring for terminally patients by advising on symptom control and psychosocial/existential issues.
- To provide extra counselling and support to relatives finding difficulties with more complex grief situations.
- To provide support and advice to the staff caring for these patients.
- To take part in multidisciplinary education relating to issues of palliative care:
  - informally at ward level
  - formal lectures
  - writing of booklets or guidelines.
- To act as a liaison between the hospital and existing hospices/home care services.
- To audit and research areas of interest such as symptom control or issues surrounding the emotional impact of dying.

The next chapter focuses on the different ways specialist palliative care teams have been set up. It also addresses the important issue of evaluation of services.

2

Setting out to meet the need

In the last chapter, we reviewed the needs of terminally ill patient and their families in the acute hospital setting. We now consider the two principal developments of the hospice movement which have sought to meet these needs: the palliative care unit and the hospital-based palliative care team. The concept of palliative care units is presented first. A brief overview is given, based on features of several units. There are only a limited number of palliative care units in the UK, which may be a result of the large number of hospice units that were built as a result of the hospice movement. However, palliative care units are more popular in other countries, particularly Canada and the US, where the charitable sector has been less involved in setting up hospices. Readers who want more information about setting up and running a unit should refer to the excellent manual by Mount *et al.* (1974).

In keeping with the theme of this book, the information given about hospital-based palliative care teams in this chapter is more comprehensive. This chapter details aspects of palliative care teams in the UK and abroad. General principles are drawn from these examples about the setting up of a palliative care team. Effective evaluation of these teams is an important and current issue. The chapter ends with discussion of current difficulties on the evaluation of these teams in the acute setting.

The palliative care unit

Within the UK, a palliative care unit represents the hospice in-patient approach within the acute hospital setting. It is a purpose-built area within the hospital. Some units are in the same grounds but are physically separate from other hospital buildings. Alternatively a separate ward or part of an existing ward may be devoted to the care of the dying. They are more commonly seen in specialist centres (for example the Royal Marsden Hospital or The Royal Heart and Chest Hospital) or where there is limited access to local hospice facilities. Often authorities have decided to invest palliative care beds into the acute hospital facility which is already available, rather than develop a separate hospice.

Most units provide a homely atmosphere where careful attention has been paid to the decor of rooms. Carpeting, soft furnishings, restful colour schemes, and the use of plants and paintings all combine to produce a therapeutic environment. Background technology is kept to a minimum. Facilities are often available to allow relatives to stay overnight, make tea and coffee, and phone other members of the family. Separate catering facilities permit flexibility in preparing and serving meals.

A high proportion of trained nursing staff is characteristic of palliative care units. This allows more time for individualized physical and psychological care for patient and families. Medical input may be through a specific consultant attached whole-time, or working part-time in addition to a hospital appointment or another palliative medicine appointment.

It is often not difficult to raise the capital to refurbish a ward or to establish a free-standing unit. However, it is much more difficult to meet running costs, particularly the salaries required to maintain a high staff/patient ratio. Inevitably, this restricts the number of beds. Palliative care units are only able to deal directly with the needs of a small minority of all patients.

A small number of beds means that an aggressive selection policy must be adopted. Otherwise, beds quickly become filled with patients who have slowly progressive disease and who cannot live at home. On the other hand, the transfer of patients who have only a matter of hours to live is upsetting to patients, family, and staff alike.

The presence of a palliative care unit may promote a 'dumping ground' philosophy in some doctors involved in acute medical care. When a dying patient presents to their service, or a patient already under their care deteriorates, they expect the patient to be moved to enable other acute patients to be admitted. If the patient is not transferred, there may be disappointment, even resentment—sentiments which detract from the patient's ongoing care in the ward. Palliative care units could therefore accentuate the idea that death must be hidden, kept apart, and not allowed to intrude on life.

In response to these concerns, some units have extended their role into the hospital by having one or two team members seeing and assessing patients on the other wards. In this way the expertise of the palliative care unit is spread into the rest of the hospital. The staff can also be used to screen patients, preventing transfer of those who are too ill to be moved or who are otherwise not appropriate for whatever other reason.

There are other ways in which staff of such units improve the care of terminally ill patients. They provide the opportunity for student nurses and junior medical staff to spend time on the unit. Unit staff are often involved in teaching programmes. Some units extend their role to provide an advisory service for the other wards. Where geographic, financial, or philosophical reasons mitigate against the establishment of a palliative care unit, the hospital-based palliative care team provides an excellent, cheaper alternative.

Hospital-based palliative care teams

As has been briefly detailed in Chapter 1, the hospital-based palliative care team in the UK has been the most recent evolution of the hospice movement. However, as long ago as 1973, Cartwright *et al.*, in their nationwide UK study of the care of the dying, stressed the importance of disseminating hospice expertise more widely into the geriatric and acute ward situation, so that all dying patients could benefit.

The first hospital-based palliative care team was established in St Luke's Hospital in New York in 1975 (O'Neil *et al.* 1992). In the UK, it was not until the founding of St Thomas' Hospital Palliative Care Team (Bates *et al.* 1981) that the need for a peripatetic team within the acute setting became more widely recognized. Despite being an advisory service, the team was able to facilitate a level of symptom control which enabled many patients to be discharged home to spend more time at home. This represented a small but significant reversal of the trend (Bates 1985). Although it is considered that people would often prefer to die at home, statistics show that the majority of deaths, even cancer deaths, still occur in the acute hospital setting despite the establishment of hospice units, and designated home care teams.

The experience of St Bartholomew's Hospital Palliative Care Team, London has been similar to that of St Thomas's Team regarding the percentage of cancer deaths occurring in the hospital setting. The Bart's team was established as a result of a study (Hockley *et al.* 1988) that looked at the needs of terminally ill patients dying on acute medical wards, and their families. Despite a desire to promote hospice/home transfer once the palliative care team was set up, 60% of patients referred to the team in 1988 still died in hospital. The reasons given were:

- unexpected deterioration while undergoing active treatment or investigations
- relatives unable to cope with home care
- late presentation precluding transfer
- waiting for transfer to hospice (Dunlop *et al.* 1989).

Bascom (1997) states the usefulness of hospital-based palliative care teams before patients are in the final stages of malignant terminal disease. A two-year education programme was set up prior to establishing a specific palliative care service in the hospital. He reports how physicians may lack the skills needed to help patients make the transition from aggressive care to care directed at more limited goals where symptom control and psychological care would be the major input. A team in Wisconsin, USA (Weissman and Griffie 1994) reports that their major referral request was for end-of-life decision-making.

O'Neil *et al.* (1992) describe three models of hospital-based palliative care teams in the US, Canada, and the UK. There is a common theme of 'financial constraints', but these services have survived with the commitment, vision, and enthusiasm of dedicated professionals. Clearly the evolution, leadership, structure, functioning, composition (see Table 2.1), and financing of teams differ from country to country and from hospital to hospital. However, the need for specialist palliative care services within the hospital cannot be denied although little rigorous evaluative research has yet to be completed.

Within the short history of specialist palliative care teams, there have been some teams that have not survived. Herxheimer *et al.* (1985)

Table 2.1 Compositions of teams: January 1991 (O'Neil *et al.* 1992)

	St Luke's	St Thomas's	Henderson
Physicians	0.65	1	1.2
Nurse clinicians	3	5	1
Social workers	1	0.8	1
Occupational therapists	0	0	0.4
Chaplains	1	0.2	0.3
Secretaries	1	1	1
Volunteer co-ordinator	1	0	1
Volunteers	40	3	6
Day centre leader	–	1	–

described the factors which can weaken the vision to establish a palliative care team and threaten its survival:

- lack of concrete committment at exective board level
- lack of funding
- lack of designated leadership
- confusion over the different roles and skills of team members
- lack of a team base
- failure in communication
- a solo team member working on their own for more than 18 months.

Unfortunately, many teams have been subject to some of these constraints. The isolation of palliative care nurse specialists is worrying.

There are now around 139 palliative care teams in the various university and district general hospitals in the UK. More than 150 other hospitals have nurse specialists working either as solo practitioners or in small groups (St Christopher's Hospice Directory 1997). The ideal model is the multidisciplinary palliative care team. However, some hospitals struggle with the financial outlay needed for such a service, particularly the medical input. There is increasing reliance on consultants being available from local hospice units.

Bennett and Corcoran (1994) have shown that hospital-based palliative care teams have an impact on palliative care services in the community. With the introduction of a palliative care team, patients were discharged more quickly and the length of stay in the community increased from 8 weeks before death to 13 weeks before death. This study confirmed that a newly established specialist palliative care team in the hospital will have implications for the activity of the local hospice as well as the local hospice home care team, owing to the heightened awareness in the hospital of the needs of dying patients and their families.

A specialist team model for children dying

Although the majority of palliative care teams based in the acute hospital work with adults, in 1984 Dr Ann Goldman established a 'symptom care team' for children with cancer at The Hospital for Sick Children, Great Ormond Street, London (GOS). Dr Goldman's vision for the new service was met with interest and enthusiasm by the oncology and haematology consultants. With this support, the basic outlines for the structure and roles of the team within the unit evolved rapidly.

Cancer in children is relatively rare. The majority of children with cancer are treated at specialist centres, and the department at GOS is the largest in the UK. The paediatric oncologists at GOS have a strong tradition of caring for the physical and psychosocial needs of their patients from diagnosis, through treatment to either cure (up to 60%) or relapse and ultimately death. For many years, this theme of continuity and total care had been provided by a team which included social workers, psychologists, play therapists, and teachers, as well as nursing and medical staff. Nevertheless, there were aspects of care which needed more attention: symptom care during treatement, terminal care, liaison, and education in paediatric palliative care.

The extremely intensive, 'high tech' nature of paediatric oncology meant that the staff in GOS tended to be tuned to the needs of patients and families on active treatment. Changing gear to palliative care for a terminally ill child on the ward was often emotionally difficult. There were also practical problems finding the time and the continuity of staff needed for such patients.

The situation of having a terminally ill child with cancer at home is so uncommon that it may occur only once or twice in the lifetime of a family practitioner, and infrequently for a general paediatrician. Home care almost inevitably provokes considerable distress and feelings of inadequacy for everyone concerned. There seemed to be a need to provide a source of experience in dealing with the psychosocial support and symptom care for the family of the child who had chosen to be at home, their primary health care team, and local hospital team.

Although there are 12 or more children's hospices in the United Kingdom (St Christopher's Hospice Information Service), their primary role has not been to provide a place for children to die but to provide a more supportive facility for families with children who have progressive, often long-term, life-threatening disease. The study of symptom control and of training in palliative care for adults has not been paralleled in paediatrics. Although some principles of hospice care apply to children, it is not enough merely to extrapolate from experience in adults (RCPCH 1997). The pharmacological handling of drugs and the types of malignancies affecting children differ from those of adults. Although children's symptoms overlap with those of adults, their relative frequency and importance will vary. The practical details of nursing care and the type of support needed by families with young children also differ from those of adults (Goldman and Baum 1994).

Evaluation of existing teams

The emergence of hospital-based palliative care teams has caused debate about the advantages and disadvantages of such teams, and their effectiveness and evaluation. Most professionals working within the acute setting appreciate the value of on-site specialist advice. However, because of financial restraints in a diminishing health care budget, palliative care teams in the acute setting cannot assume that this appreciation will translate into ongoing financial support. If such teams are to be developed in the acute setting rigorous evaluation of their effectiveness will be required.

Advantages of palliative care teams

One of the main advantages of hospital-based palliative care teams is the dissemination of hospice expertise to those who do not want to die in a hospice or for whom a non-malignant disease precludes transfer to a hospice facility. By serving as a resource for other professionals, such teams make hospice relevant to all terminally ill patients and their families, not just to cancer patients. Good symptom control can be transferred from the hospice unit to the acute hospital setting (Ellershaw *et al.* 1995). One of the main reasons for setting up the team at St Thomas' Hospital was to help with the symptom control of terminally ill patients and thereby enable such patients to be at home for longer periods and even to be able to die in their own home. With an on-site palliative care team, symptom control and appropriate care can be available from an earlier point in the disease process, without waiting until the end stage of an illness. This can often pre-empt patients and families having to face a crisis situation during the dying phase.

The palliative care team represents a visible standard of care. It is more difficult for a sub-optimal practice of care for the dying to be practised if ward staff are being reminded and supported by a specialist team. This can revitalize the care of the dying, acting as a counterbalance to the upward spiral of pressure on ward teams. Palliative care teams can help ward teams take the time and have the satisfaction of thinking through basic problems, and seeing this translated into better care of the dying. These teams also provide continuity of care for patients and their families, countering the disruption of staff rotation on the wards.

The palliative care team can improve the knowledge and skills of symptom control and psychosocial care by teaching on the medical and nursing school curricula and also by acting as 'role models'. It is difficult to teach these skills didactically. However, with a multidisciplinary team of specialists these skills can be passed on and reinforced in the setting of the acute hospital ward.

The palliative care team within the acute setting can be a bridge to a hospice home-care service or hospice unit. The ambassadorial role can benefit both hospital and hospice service; keeping each up-to-date with the most recent change in technologies and techniques. It is important to encourage a balanced view about what each service has to offer. Hospices and hospitals can promote expert, compassionate care and advice for the dying which is appropriate to their situation.

Disadvantages of palliative care teams

Bates *et al.* (1981) stressed that the presence of a hospital-based palliative care team can cause potential confusion over responsibility of care. However much a team member is involved with a patient, the responsibility of care rests firmly with the consultant in charge of the patient. It should be a very rare exception that the primary team hands over the responsibility. In some cases this happens but most palliative care teams have no authority to admit patients. Constant written communication in the notes is vital to keep the referring team as involved as possible.

There is a danger that a team which is meant to improve the standard of care for the dying in hospital becomes the agent for doing the work. The ward team then have an excuse not to be involved. This does not happen when the staff of a ward are motivated to care for the dying , but it can easily happen when the incentive to care is taken away because the patient relates to the specialist team instead of the primary team. Team members must act as role models rather than take over care. If you do not ensure that ward staff are involved with patient and family interviews, then there is a danger of suppressing an interest in 'care of the dying', and de-skilling of ward staff.

One of the difficulties of working on a palliative care team is the compromise that is sometimes necessary. Although the palliative care team is there to represent hospice principles, there are times when you cannot deliver the care that would be possible within the atmosphere of the hospice setting. It is particularly distressing when compromise is needed to placate the primary team and ensure future referrals rather than 'holding out' on an issue for the sake of the principle.

A palliative care team within the hospital may experience fewer deaths compared to colleagues working in hospices. However, the work is no less demanding. Factors which can cause considerable tension include

- not having total management over patients
- the different philosophies of truth-telling which staff operate
- the frustration of waiting for the ward team to carry out suggestions.

It may seem easier to do the task yourself but although there are some situations where this is appropriate, it should not become the 'norm', otherwise the team's potential will be diminished.

Within the hospital environment, the palliative care team is often working in an atmosphere that seems highly charged. Team members have to constantly check the appropriateness of further active treatment, understand the patient's wishes and decide whether to challenge decisions made by the referring team. This can give the sensation of 'swimming against the tide' of normal hospital practice. Working in the atmosphere of the acute setting can heighten anxiety, which can sometimes diminish your effectiveness with patients and their families. In hospital there is considerable overt pressure on beds which can often make you feel pressurized into transferring a patient inappropriately, or face the difficult situation of having to readmit a patient when there are no beds available.

The difficult and challenging situations posed in hospitals often attract strong personalities on to a palliative care team. It is important for team personnel to be able to withstand these pressures, but this should be through skill and expertise rather than a overly strong ego. This is not easy because the roles of team members are less well defined than the normal roles of health care workers within the hospital or hospice setting.

Effectiveness and evaluation of services

Given the difficulties, the question arises whether the needs of the dying can be met in hospital. It has been argued that acute wards are not suitable for terminally ill patients because the necessary standard of care cannot be provided (NWTRHA 1987). This argument could seriously weaken support for plans to set up a team. There is now some data which confirm that palliative care teams are effective at relieving symptoms (Bruera *et al.* 1989; Ellershaw *et al.* 1995). Further research into the efficacy and cost-effectiveness of palliative care teams' is important but is also an extremely complex task. There are several detailed evaluations currently under way which may provide more definite answers.

The National Hospice Study (Greer *et al.* 1986) provided indirect evidence in support of the advisory role performed by palliative care teams. It was the first major study to compare palliative care in oncology units with hospice care and hospice–home-care. The results showed that the different settings fared equally well; hospice units provided somewhat better control of pain and other symptoms, and relatives were more satisfied with hospice care. Unfortunately one of the major limitations of this study was the fact that patients selected which service they wanted and would therefore be generally satisfied with the care received. However, the study did not report the observation that the quality of conventional hospital care improved during the study. The improvements occurred because hosptial care-givers were under review, which motivated them to improve standards (D.S. Greer, personal communication). This suggests that heightening awareness of deficiencies in care, for example through the presence of a palliative care team, can stimulate change.

Parkes' longitudinal study (1985) suggested that education can improve pain control in hospital. In the initial study, the small number of hospice patients experiencing severe pain prior to death contrasted sharply with the hospital experience. During a 10 year period, pain control in the hospitals near St Christopher's Hospice, London improved to the extent that there was no longer any significant difference. Parkes felt that the improvement represented an effect of the hospice's education programme. Many doctors and nurses from the study hospitals had attended teaching sessions. Although patient care improved, Parkes found that the care of relatives was less satisfactory in hospital. He suggested that attention to relatives' needs was difficult to translate into the hospital setting.

Indirect evidence indicates hospital palliative care teams can improve relatives' care. We reviewed letters of complaint received by the hospital administration at St Bartholomew's Hospital. Before the introduction of the palliative care team, 8% of the total number of complaints came from relatives of dying patients. These complaints declined steadily to less than 1% after 4 years of the team's being in operation (Hockley *et al.* 1988).

McQuay and Moore (1994) state that randomized control trials are mandatory for evaluating palliative care services in the acute setting. They go on to say that 'the provision of a service is much more subjective than the provision of an intervention'. Randomized control trials are currently seen as the 'gold standard'. McWhinney *et al.* (1994) discuss the unique ethical and methodological difficulties of using randomization to evaluate palliative care services. The UCLA evaluation (Wales *et al.*, 1983) was one of the first randomized control trials of hospice care conducted. Although it was not conclusive, the study looked at pain and symptom control, mood, functional status, family satisfaction, choice of place of death, and carer's morbidity during bereavement. Unfortunately, the large number of well-established palliative care services/teams within the acute setting have made it difficult to carry out a randomized control trial of this type of service.

One hospital in Southampton, England (Davies, personal communication) tried to randomize the intervention for terminally ill patients to two different surgical wards. One ward had the input of the palliative care team. The 'control' ward had normal input from the surgical team. Unfortunately the study was abandoned because staff on the 'control' ward transferred patients with complex problems to the ward where the palliative care team was working. The rotation of doctors from the 'experimental' to the 'control' ward would also inevitably contaminate the sample.

There is now some data to confirm evidence that specialist palliative care intervention can be effective (Bruera *et al.* 1989, Ellershaw *et al.* 1995, Abraham *et al.* 1996, Jarvis *et al.* 1996, McQuillan *et al.* 1996). Most confirm the importance of the educational aspect of a palliative care service within the hospital. The study by Ellershaw *et al.* (1995) shows that a hospital palliative care team is effective at improving symptom control, facilitating the understanding of diagnosis and prognosis as well as contributing to the appropriate placement of patients in hospice, home or nursing home. Bruera *et al.* (1989) concluded that the presence of the pain and symptom control team resulted in some changes in the pattern of care, particularly the continued improvement in pain assessment by nurses and the pattern of prescribing by the residents.

Conclusive evidence about the other aspects of hospital-based palliative care teams must be obtained to support the increasing financial outlay for these teams. This involves examining the impact of the team on all aspects of care, not only in relation to pain and symptom control but also continuing education, staff attitudes towards the dying and end-of-life decision-making. Clearly, the research designs for such studies need to take into account the different hospital situations, as well as build on the experience and methodologies of earlier studies. A 3 year study taking place at the Western General Hospital, Edinburgh (WGH) is using a quasi-experimental method comparing surgical units in different university hospitals—the unit at WGH with the on-site palliative care team is the experimental arm of the study. The study will compare specific patient and relative outcomes. It will also examine the attitudes and knowledge of medical and nursing staff, and attempt to estimate cost-effectiveness.

As can be seen from the above, most of the research evaluating hospital-based palliative care teams has concentrated on interventions that benefit patient care rather than on the cost of achieving the benefits (Normand 1996). This is an important issue for palliative care especially given the current financial problems facing health care (Robbins 1997). A recent randomized control trial looking at the cost-effectiveness of a district-wide service which coordinated the care of patients with cancer (Raftery *et al.* 1996) reported that the costs incurred by the coordination group were significantly less than those of the control group. The coordinated group used significantly fewer in-patient days, which contributed to the mean cost per coordinated patient being almost half that of the control group patients. Although the intervention was not made by a palliative care team, the roles of the coordinators were similar to the roles of team members in hospitals. Weissman and Griffie (1994) argue that there is poor coordination of the care of the dying in the acute hospital setting without an on-site specialist palliative care service.

Some guidelines for planning a palliative care team

There is no single blueprint for establishing a hospital-based palliative care team. However, there are general principles which may help to guide you.

Someone with vision and commitment

Most teams have started from the enthusiasm and insight of individual doctors or nurses who have been moved by the special needs of the terminally ill in hospital. These individuals have often had contact with the hospice movement. This has fuelled the desire to disseminate principles and practice of hospice care back into the acute hospital setting.

Other health professionals may interpret the proposals for a palliative care team as an attempt at 'empire building'. It is vital, therefore, that at least one person has the necessary vision and stamina to survive the inevitable delays, frustrations, and setbacks that characterize the planning phase. It may well take several years from the inception of a project to a team becoming operational. The teams that are most likely to last are those that have been well researched and planned so that the funders are well informed and enthused. It cannot be stressed enough that the hospital administration must be in favour of such a project if it is not to fail.

The above describes a 'top down' approach and will generally involve someone at quite a high level (i.e. consultant or director of nursing) to instigate the idea and gain support for the project. Usually, both a consultant and director of nursing will need to be involved in order to convince those at hospital board level.

Occasionally, palliative care teams have been established as the result of regional adminstrative directives. Although this would sound like a 'top down' approach, there is often not the commitment at board level to see the project through. A lone nurse specialist or palliative medicine physician is put into a job so that the board are seen to be doing the right thing. There may be more success for a doctor in this situation than a nurse specialist, but in either case it will be extremely taxing. The person may be a visionary and have considerable palliative care experience but if they are not part of the power structure of the hospital then there will be an uphill battle to achieve the commitment of support and the funding for a multidisciplinary team.

Identifying the needs

Although the weight of evidence about unmet needs of patients, families, and staff caring for the dying in the acute hospital setting is considerable, sadly it may still be necessary to convince some administrators and other influential members of staff that the terminally ill do not receive adequate care. Several people have undertaken projects to assess their local situation (Hockley *et al.* 1988, Hockley 1989, Simpson 1991, Greenhill 1996, McQuillan *et al.* 1996). Projects can take from 3 weeks to 6 months, depending on resources available. There are a number of simple tools that can be used. Several studies have used research to identify the needs of the dying patient and family in order to facilitate the creation of a team (Hockley *et al.* 1988; Simpson 1991). This certainly helps to focus the attention of managers and senior clinicians on the problems. The results can also be used as a baseline to show improved care in pain, symptom control, communication once the specialist palliative care team has become established.

The authors would like to stress how useful it is to collect baseline data prior to setting up a service. Quite apart from the collection of data, these projects can improve the acceptance of the palliative care team in the early operational phase. Hospital staff will become familiar with the investigator before he or she begins operating in an advisory capacity as a member of the palliative care team.

Identifying services already involved in meeting needs

Some effort should be made to meet with general practitioners, district nurses, hospice staff, home care teams, bereavement groups, and other services which are providing care for the terminally ill within the district. This is particularly important if a palliative care team is to be funded by the NHS. Many of these other services will be funded charitably and may feel their existence is threatened by the new service. Concerns may also be eased by allowing existing services to be represented on a planning committee.

Even with good preparation, difficulties will arise because of perceived and actual similarities in roles. Doctors may find it difficult to accept that specialist nurses will provide advice about medications. Social workers are likely to be unsettled by the appointment of nurse specialists who have a specific counselling role. Doctors and nurse specialists in radiotherapy and oncology units may also feel threatened. Usually, exisiting non-palliative care services feel threatened out of ignorance of what can be achieved with a specialist palliative care team. The temptation is to appoint experienced, well-meaning oncology nurses who are less threatening to medical oncologists for example. However, those being appointed to the team must be specialists in palliative care—they must have something to offer the various wards and departments.

Mobilizing support

There may be little difficulty in finding people willing to lend moral and practical support to setting up a team. If the visionaries are not part of the administration then it will be essential to set up a working party to oversee the project. Sometimes a working party is established prior to any specific post being advertised. At other times, such a group can add momentum to the acceptance of a team. A working party should mostly comprise people who are in favour of the project and who have influence with the hospital administration. It should be fully multidisciplinary including interested consultants and nurse managers, an adminstrator, chaplain(s), social work, pharmacists, psychologist/psychiatrist, etc. If there are one or two influential consultants in appropriate specialties (ie oncology, anaesthetics) who are unsure about, or who may be antagonistic to, the concept of a palliative care team, then it is often helpful to get their participation rather than have them undermine the project.

Some staff will have negative feelings about a proposed team. If 'new' money is seen to be diverted to terminal care at a time when funding of established services is being cut back, then bitterness will add to any sense of threat and criticism. Opponents may actively undermine the team by spreading misinformation and then witholding patient or family referrals. Several teams have felt that more time should have been devoted to addressing these feelings during the planning phase.

Finding funds

A hospital-based palliative care team is reasonably inexpensive to run, as it operates within the existing hospital structure. Expenses can sometimes be shared throughout a number of specialties. However, insufficient funds frequently limit the size of a team. If team members are being expected to negotiate for funds then it is important to expect negotiations to take a long time, and to be punctuated by frequent setbacks.

Ideally, the salaries of team members should be provided by the local hospital administration but in the UK this is rarely realized in the first instance. Occasionally, the regional health administration will make funding available to implement directives. It may be possible to obtain short-term funding from this source for researching needs.

More commonly, short-term funding has to be obtained from legacies, or charitable trusts such as Macmillan Cancer Relief. Drug companies have sometimes given financial support. Ultimately, health authorities or the hospital administration need to take over after two or three years. By securing charity funding for each post, new members can gradually be added to the team. This dovetails nicely with the increasing workload which can often be sufficient for one person to cope with during the first 18 months.

The availability of money from non-hospital sources may make it difficult to gauge the true level of adminstrative support. The administration may pay lip-service to the principles of terminal care while the money is forthcoming. The true depth and sincerity of support will only become apparent when the short-term funding expires. A lack of concrete financial support was instrumental in the collapse of the Charing Cross Hospital Team (Herxheimer *et al.* 1985). Fortunately, this team is now fully operational again.

Planning for the practical needs of a palliative care team

Some thought needs to be given to the name of the team as this can affect how the team is perceived. One team was criticized for being called a 'special care team'—other staff wondered why the team was so 'special'. Two clinical nurse specialists were identified as 'care of the dying sister'. Only patients who were actually dying were referred and the nurses felt their skills in palliative care were underutilized.

The titles of teams have changed over the last 10 years. With palliative medicine becoming recognized in the UK as a specialty in its own right, the term palliative care team has replaced terminal care support teams or support care team. However, many patients and their families are unfamiliar with the word 'palliative' and considerable explanation may be needed. In the past, the title 'support care team' was useful as the initials could be interchanged with 'symptom control team'. The flexibility allowed the former name to be used to convey a sense of comfort to patients with psychosocial problems, whereas the latter name reassured patients with symptoms who were hesitant about the psychological connotation of 'support'.

The provision of adequate office space is paramount. The physical environment of the office can have important effects on team morale and stress. Space is very often at a premium in existing hospitals, and office space is likely to be small and cramped. An increase in the number of team members will make the effect of office size more pronounced. Often one has to accept any office to begin with but this should not be shared with another facility. After other team members have been appointed, it is easier to pester the authorities for better accommodation.

An office which is geographically distant from hospital wards will create a sense of isolation, particularly if there are no other full-time members. Maintaining a profile on the wards will be difficult. Consequently, hospital staff will be less familiar with the team, and fewer referrals will be made. The prospect of a significant journey will deter retreat to the relative peace of the office after a stressful experience. An office by a busy corridor will increase contact with other hospital staff but may not allow privacy for team meetings.

It is important to ensure an adequate number of phones. In general, there should be one phone line per team member. In reality this is generally not possible but the team should have at least three phone lines, especially if one line is to be used for a fax machine. A direct line which bypasses the hospital switchboard is helpful for calls to relatives and out-patients. Where teams are part of a cancer centre that covers a whole region, the capability to make long-distance calls will facilitate liaison with other teams and hospices. An answerphone will improve communication, particularly if there is no secretary to take calls during the day. Some relatives appreciate being able to leave a message after hours when there is no 24 hour service.

Office and administration costs of the team have to be fully integrated into the hospital financial system or the team given a realistic budget. Because the hospital administration often has considerable help from charities to fund the salaries, they can often be persuaded to provide a computer, filing cabinets, and other office furniture.

There are two other steps which are essential to the planning process: developing job descriptions, and selecting team members. Because of the importance of these related steps, we have devoted the next chapter to them.

3

Selecting team members

Palliative care teams have developed a variety of responses to meet the needs of dying patients and their families in different hospitals. In almost all palliative care teams, clinical nurse specialists form the backbone of the service. One or more doctors, a social worker, a psychologist, a secretary, and the clergy may also be represented in many different combinations. Volunteers, social work assistants, bereavement counsellors, and health visitors also work as an integral part of some teams. The efficiency of the multidisciplinary team coupled with the presence of specialist medical input is needed to maximize credibility among hospital consultants.

It is not uncommon for teams to start with one member; indeed, many small hospitals have only a single nurse specialist (Morris 1981). For the purpose of compiling data about palliative care services, solo nurse specialists are not counted as 'teams'. It is important to recognize that nurse specialists in palliative care cannot operate effectively in isolation, and need a network of colleagues—nursing, medical, and other—to provide additional advice and support.

Each putative member of a new team should have a clearly defined role. Clear-cut job descriptions are essential for establishing the criteria used in the selection process. Applicants require guidelines on which to base their decision to apply for the post, and members of the interview panel must have an adequate understanding of the job in order to assess the suitability of applicants. Once staff are in post, a realistic understanding of each person's role will make for greater team effectiveness and harmony.

The following descriptions of the tasks, responsibilities, and skills required of team members are based on the collective experiences of various teams visited and interviewed by the authors. These profiles are not intended to be prescriptive but can be used as a basis for planning job descriptions. Where possible, these descriptions should be supplemented by a visit to teams working in similar circumstances before deciding on the best formula for local needs.

Clinical nurse specialists

The role of the clinical nurse specialist is now more widely accepted and understood than it was in the early 1980s when palliative care teams were first being created. As its name suggests, the nurse is a specialist in a specific area. The fact that there is now a specialist register (Colquhoun and Dougan 1997) for nurses working in palliative care shows how far nurse specialization in palliative care has developed in the last five years. However, just because a nurse's name is on the register doesn't necessarily confirm *clinical expertise* in palliative care. It is important to examine the areas from which the clinical experience has been gained.

The recent Calman–Hine report on the development of cancer services in the UK has advocated site-specific specialization in cancer treatment. An increasing number of nurse specialists fulfil a role as site-specific nurse specialists within the clinical oncology team, for example breast care nurses, etc. It is important that nurse specialists in palliative care are well skilled and experienced in their own field. If this is not the case there is a potential for confusion over roles.

Interestingly, many nurses applying for hospital-based nurse specialist palliative care posts have not worked in the hospice setting. Many nurses want to work in hospices because they are dissatisfied with the quality of nursing dying patients in hospitals; they often do not want to return to stress and frustration of the acute setting. Clinical nurse specialists have been able to work effectively in palliative care teams with minimum prior hospice experience but usually within the context of an established team. If a nurse is being asked to set up a team in the hospital then it is vital to have considerable clinical hospice experience.

In situations where there is a solo nurse specialist in a district general hospital it is important that the role is clearly understood and is precisely defined in the job description. Even though a nurse might have considerable oncology experience, it does not automatically make him/her a clinical nurse specialist in palliative care. The days have gone when a nurse specialist can be all things to all people. A clear concise job description is vitally important.

The majority of nurse specialists working on palliative care teams are employed full-time; nurses working part-time usually complement full-time colleagues. A nurse specialist will often be the main coordinator by virtue of being the only full-time team member. In larger teams, the majority of team members will be nurse specialists, which parallels the fact that nurses are the main care-givers within the hospital setting. In many ways the role of the nurse specialist is more blurred than for other palliative care team members. In general the doctor will focus on symptom control problems and the patient/family understanding about the diagnosis and prognosis. The social worker and psychologist likewise will have important skills to help with family issues, bereavement, and psychosocial difficulties. The nurse specialist's boundaries are less defined. This is partly because of the skills they should have in symptom control and psychosocial care but also because of the intuitive learned experience of nursing dying patients and their families in general.

In the past most nurse specialists in palliative care would have had prior experience as ward sisters or district nursing sisters. Now, however, this may not be the case. The role of ward sister in particular has become more managerial than clinical over the last few years. Nonetheless, having experience of organizing and running a ward can be an advantage in understanding the pressures of ward life and the importance of interacting with consultants and senior medical staff. A district nurse or health visitor qualification may be an absolute requirement if members of the team are to work in the community. This qualification confers the experience of planning discharges or helping with bereavement which can be an added bonus to a team.

If there is no specialist palliative care experience, then working in a hospice for a short period in order to build confidence on symptom control issues and speaking about dying with patients and their families can be extremely useful prior to taking on a nurse specialist post in the acute setting. In a small survey of the first palliative care teams created in the 1980s, two thirds of palliative care teams felt that more hospice experience would have been beneficial in reducing the stress associated with advising hospital doctors and general practitioners about symptom control. Others felt that, although working in hospice provided considerable experience in symptom management, it did not prepare them for the major stresses of trying to apply these principles within the hospital setting (Hockley, unpublished data).

Nurses working on a hospital palliative care team are under different pressures from their colleagues working in hospices or in the community. Clinical nurse specialists within the acute setting may not have to face the same number of deaths as their colleagues working in a hospice. However, the necessary skills required are probably at least as demanding if not more so, especially if they are working alone. Many referrals to a hospital specialist team for palliative care advice involve difficult symptom control issues. At least one of the nurses on the team must be confident and skilled in this area if the team is going to be able to gain the respect of the referring consultants. Nurses who had prior hospice experience felt this had been essential for enabling them to undertake the advisory and teaching roles.

The specialist expertise for the job in question must be well grounded. If the hospital has identified a need for advice/teaching on symptom control then the first person appointed to build a team must be expert in this area. If, however, there is greater emphasis for improving psychosocial support then these skills must be present. It is no good to think that team members are going to learn on the job. Being thrown as a specialist into an advisory position is a recipe for disaster if the person employed does not have the appropriate expertise.

Job descriptions are now well documented for nurse specialists in palliative care. Given the hierarchical structure of acute hospital services, accountability and responsibility for the nurse specialist will frequently involve senior nurses and other administrators who are physically remote from the team. This can create considerable stress if solo nurse specialists are unable to get support and a degree of clinical supervision from other palliative care specialists nearby. In an isolated area where there is no local hospice the hospital management must be committed to promoting the principles of palliative care and fully support the nurse specialist post that has been created. The job is hard enough without the lack of managerial support.

Where a hospital is in a fortunate position to be able to support more than one nurse specialist in palliative care, it is important that the expertise, experience, and skill mix of the nurse specialists are considered. A good mixture of clinical skills both within palliative care nursing and other related fields, teaching experience, computer literacy, and experience in audit and/or research can produce an extremely effective team.

There are considerable variations about whether palliative care nurse specialists wear uniform. A uniform has the advantage of immediately clarifying the status of the nurse to the patient, family, or other staff. Wearing everyday clothes and a clear name badge identifying status, on the other hand, has the advantage of emphasizing the advocate role of the specialist on behalf of the patient and family. The latter is probably now the most common approach. Either way, maintaining a distinction between the ward nursing staff and the nurse specialist facilitates the teaching and advisory roles without taking over nursing procedures, although there are times when providing practical help is necessary.

Teaching plays an important part for the nurse on a palliative care team. Having the skill and enthusiasm to pass on knowledge can be an asset to the daily practice of the nurse specialist. Quite apart from educating other carers (see chapter 7), teaching can have a recharging effect in what may otherwise be, at times, an emotionally draining job. Both informal and formal teaching should represent a significant proportion of the role.

Career pathways for the nurse specialist in palliative care may appear restricted, especially if the nurse has limited nursing experience and only a general nursing qualification. Increasingly, specific qualifications are required in order to change the direction of one's job, for example going into the community or into teaching. The nurse specialist is in a unique position, having gained considerable experience in the care of the dying and their families. Much of this experience becomes intuitive and needs to be looked at more critically through reflection and possibly research. Obviously full-time research is open to nurse specialists who have already done a first degree. However, funding is difficult to get, especially to ensure comparability with a nurse specialist's salary. A step into management, such as a director of nursing in a hospice, might not be possible except for someone who is keen to study for an MBA. There are an increasing number of strategic planning or audit positions in palliative care.

Doctors

The first wave of palliative care teams within the acute setting were all set up with either a full-time or part-time doctor. More recently within the UK, nurse specialists have been put into post often without the appropriate medical back-up. Palliative care teams who do no have a doctor as part of the team may find that they lack a degree of credibility, particularly with medical staff. Non-medical team members will potentially be more stressed by having to carry the responsibility of advising on medical issues.

In 1987 palliative medicine was recognized by the Royal College of Physicians in the UK as a specialty in its own right. This has made a career in the specialty more attractive. With a specialist registrar training post it is often possible to get experience of working on a hospital-based palliative care team alongside experience within the local hospice. However, any permanent full-time or part-time medical post would commonly be at consultant/senior lecturer level. Such posts are still often difficult to establish because of funding. Some teams in the past have had an interested consultant available on a voluntary basis; the doctor usually attends the main multidisciplinary meeting each week. This arrangement may work well in a small hospital, particularly when financial constraints limit the size of the team, but will prove unsatisfactory if the doctor is not available when needed or is not able to attend team meetings. The resultant stress on the other team members can be greater than the stress of having no doctor at all. The difficulty of this arrangement was exemplified by the Charing Cross Hospital Terminal Care Support Team (Herxheimer *et al.* 1985). There is a trend for consultants from nearby hospice units to allocate one or two sessions for supporting solo nurse specialists, for example seeing patients on the ward at their request.

Maguire (1985) suggested that there may be some advantage in working part-time. More time is available to pursue other clinical interests, which reduces the stress inherent in terminal care. This suggestion should be given careful consideration, given that the team doctor's role is to advise rather than take over care. Specialist training in other fields, including working in a hospice, will have involved the doctor exercising responsibility for patients. It can be extremely difficult for a doctor to relinquish this. Negotiating every investigation or change in medication can be disheartening and humiliating, especially if the primary team declines to follow suggestions. The credibility of the doctor will depend on being able to control difficult symptoms, especially when the doctors of the referring team have strong emotional ties with a terminally ill patient. If the patient is a personal friend or a prominent citizen, the referring team will closely monitor what is done. If the team doctor is able to help, barriers will be broken and the team will be more widely accepted and used. This effect can even overcome the barrier of the team doctor not being a 'specialist'.

Doctors working with palliative care teams come from a wide variety of specialist backgrounds: radiotherapy, oncology, anaesthetics, general medicine, psychiatry, clinical pharmacology, and general practice. Although these backgrounds are all quite different, the common denominator which appears to draw the person into palliative care team work within the hospital is the deeply felt concern for improving the quality of life for terminally ill patients and their families.

Providing expertise on difficult symptom control problems is one of the specific responsibilities on the doctor as a member of the palliative care team (see Table 3.1). Nurses can gain the experience necessary to advise on medication changes for many problems, but this experience may not always take into account subtle changes that may be necessary to avoid patients developing side-effects as a result of other medical conditions. Situations may arise that require an unusual use of a drug such as lignocaine or flecainide for deafferentation pain. It is far easier for a referring team to accept explanation and reassurance from the doctor on the team. If the referral has come from a medical or surgical ward, the doctor may provide insight into the rarer manifestations of cancer and cancer treatment.

The medical management of non-malignant conditions, such as manipulating diuretics and vasodilators in heart-failure, may require the specific expertise of the doctor. Reviewing investigations for difficult diagnostic problems or reviewing the response to radiation and chemotherapy, especially if chemotherapy is being administered by non-oncologists, can be a useful adjunct to the medical role. Medical and surgical teams often have problems when diagnostic and therapeutic possibilities are not clear cut or include high risk/low benefit options. The palliative care doctor can help clarify the debate on the medical management or end-of-life decisions. If the doctor avoids this respons-ibility, greater stress is imposed on the other team members but there is always the need to balance the fact that the team's involvement is by *invitation* of the referring team. The greater the respect from the referring team the easier it is to participate in such discussions. This respect can take many months before it materializes, partly because referring consultants do not have a continual flow of patients to be referred to the team.

End-of-life decision-making may not only be an issue for the referring

Table 3.1 Specific reasons for having a part-time/full time doctor on the team

---

- To provide expertise in symptom control with more complex symptom problems
- To debate the medical management of patients who are terminally ill from either cancer or non-malignant cause
- To help clarify difficulties associated with end-of-life decision-making with the referring team, patients, and relatives
- To help educate medical students, junior doctors and nurses, etc.
- To present complex cases alongside other senior doctors so as to heighten the awareness of palliative care within the acute setting
- To stimulate the impetus for clinical research and publication within the team

---

team. On some occasions an anxious relative may need further time to discuss and debate decisions. Even if the referring team and the patient have come to terms with the decision, the relative will often need further explanation. Nurse specialists can spend considerable time in resolving fears but some patients or relatives can find it very helpful if the specialist palliative care doctor can lend medical authority to the situation. This requires careful collaboration which emphasizes rather than undermines the status of the nurse specialist.

The non-medical members of the team will find it helpful if the doctor can provide some understanding about how doctors make decisions. Non-medical staff are not always aware of the unique stresses faced by the medical profession and this may lead to misinterpretation of decisions about patient management. The effectiveness of the team will be enhanced if their anger about a particular doctor's decision is redirected into sympathetic understanding (not to be confused with agreement).

It is important that the teaching role of the doctor is balanced with the necessary clinical workload. The amount of teaching that is possible will depend on how many sessions are available. With the clinical workload of a palliative care team being rather unpredictable it is important that any teaching commitments are made in the light of this unpredictability. The doctor will often play a major role in the teaching of medical students and junior doctors. At consultant level, forums such as medical and surgical grand rounds may be used. This not only helps to heighten the awareness of palliative care amongst senior doctors but also enables a subtle way of exposing them to new ideas within a forum that is familiar and comfortable. Where possible, other members of the team should be involved to exemplify the multidisciplinary approach.

The impetus for clinical research and publication may need to come from the doctor on the team although this is by no means exclusive. Nurses are becoming more aware of the importance of contributing to palliative care journals within the specialty of palliative care and more journals are seeking nursing contributions. The doctor can often be involved with research, either within the palliative care team or working in collaboration with local hospices.

The doctor, and other team members, should be alert to the way in which the interest of the doctor may impose on and limit the functioning of the team. An anaesthetist might emphasize the role of nerve blocks for pain to the extent that the team functions predominantly as a pain clinic. Involvement with patients who have other symptoms or psychosocial needs could decrease. A strong interest in acute and chronic benign pain may also be unbalancing. The relationships of the doctor will also be important. A doctor who is also attached to oncology or radiotherapy may receive a number of referrals from these specialities. However, referrals from physicians, and surgeons may be reduced because of a fear that their patient may be 'taken over'. The converse may apply if the doctor is not respected by oncology colleagues.

Funding for the medical input into the specialist palliative care team can be difficult. If the team relies on a specialist registrar, its stability and morale will be threatened by the frequent turn-around of the various doctors on rotation. A permanent post, whether part-time or full-time, at senior lecturer/consultant level is vital for most designated cancer centres in order to influence both teaching and clinical aspects of palliative medicine. Newly emerging teams have gone to charitable organizations such as Macmillan Cancer Relief in order to secure the first three or five years' funding of a senior medical post on the team. After that it is the responsibility of either the university (for senior lecturer) or part university/part hospital. The hospital NHS Trust of course is reliant on the 'purchasers'.

Secretary

A secretary for a specialist palliative care team can be one of the most pivotal positions of the team and certainly maintains a sense of continuity in the hive of activity often associated with a small team. Even if there is only a part-time secretary, a solo nurse specialist can be released to use the skills he or she was appointed for. Many teams nowadays use computer software in order to collect data on patient referrals and audit. Although very useful, this is time consuming and takes team members away from the clinical area if there is no secretary to help.

Ideally, a secretary should be part of the team. This often has to be on a part-time basis, with only a small number of large multidisciplinary teams being able to maintain a full-time secretary. A secretary may be a volunteer but this can prove difficult because of the unpredictable nature of the work load. The secretary will be responsible for maintaining team correspondence, files, and records of patient and team statistics, preparing reports, and typing lecture notes/acetates. Communication with primary care teams, other palliative care teams and hospices, patients and their relatives can be enhanced with the personal touch of a secretary answering the telephone rather than an impersonal, potentially intimidating answerphone. Referrals may be received by the secretary, which avoids team members being interupted from what may be an important conversation with a patient.

In some situations the secretary has acted as an important liaison for relatives, especially after the family member has died. Being able to pick up the phone and speak to an understanding voice from a team previously involved in the care can be an enormous support. It is not every secretary who has this ability and some would not expect it to be part of their job description. If a secretary took on this role over and above their normal secretarial duties then they would need to be supported and recognized by the whole team. Nonetheless, a part-counselling role can help make the secretary's role more satisfying given that so much of his or her time is spent alone in the office.

Psychologist

There is now more recognition for the role of psychologists working in teaching or district general hospitals. Their professional alignment with specialties such as oncology, neurology, and chronic pain clinics is already well accepted. A psychologist being a member of a palliative care team is an exciting venture and is becoming more common. It is most likely to happen when the palliative care team is closely linked to a specialty that has a psychologist who can be shared. Whether the psychologist is a member of the core team or has links on a limited sessional basis will depend on funding, and the assessment of needs within the context of the palliative care team set-up. Where there is the luxury of having someone dedicated to the team full-time or part-time, it can make a considerable difference (Lassauniere 1994).

The psychosocial aspects of palliative care have been traditionally incorporated into the holistic approach by those specialists working on a palliative care team. Psychologists can help with some of the more difficult situations either before death has occurred or with families after a bereavement. Traditionally there has been little funding for anything other than a part-time psychologist. A limited number of sessions per week automatically limits clinical involvement to only one or two patients or families at any one time.

A psychologist attached to a team can support team members in other ways. In some teams, the psychologist provides personal supervision, especially for some nurse specialists. Obviously this depends not only on the psychologist's perceived role but also on those seeking personal supervision. Probably one of the most complex aspects of any team is that of its dynamics (see chapter 6). Different personalities working in a highly charged atmosphere of palliative care within the acute hospital brings its own pressures. Some teams will use a psychologist to help them examine team dynamics, especially if internal problems exist. Stress and 'burnout' are indeed dangers of this work, neither of which is easily recognized by the individuals involved.

Social worker

Over the last 10 years, the social workers' role has changed considerably. Traditionally it has been to help families with social, emotional, or practical problems. However, within the UK, the Community Care Act (1990) has meant that social workers have a major role in organizing care and placement for the elderly. This is especially true for social workers working within the acute hospital setting. The severe restrictions in the social worker's role have made other opportunities very attractive. Social work posts in palliative care teams are often inundated with applicants.

Social work has always been seen as an important complementary role within the hospice movement. Most hospices traditionally have a social worker. If there is no specialist social worker attached to a palliative care team then the team members liaise with the individual social worker allocated to the primary team caring for the patient. Even when there is a specialist social worker, if the primary team social worker is already seeing a patient and wishes to stay involved then they will remain the key social worker. Teams that are large enough to have a social worker allocated, or specifically appointed, are fortunate. Often the initial funding has to be sought through a charity prior to being taken up by the Trust/hospital. Only 10% of palliative care teams have their own dedicated social worker (St Christopher's Hospice Information Service, London). The Association of Hospice Social Workers in the UK is a useful source of information regarding job descriptions.

The question of appointing a social worker needs to be considered within the wider context. Because funding for planning new or additional services is so limited, it is important to see what other specialist resources are already in place.

- Is there enough specialist expertise within the social work department not to require a social worker on the team?

- Can a social worker be shared with a local hospice?
- Will the team be better complemented with a psychologist and use the social worker allocated to the primary team caring for the patient?
- What other specialist social worker in palliative care is there in the region?

The answers to these questions will vary for each team. The role of the social worker is often not considered earlier enough in the team's evolution. Even if not officially paid as a member of the specialist palliative care services, an interested social worker will often help to supervise a lone clinical nurse specialist and provide other support.

The social worker assesses and advises on the psychological, emotional and social problems of patients and their family. The assessment of family attitudes and resources forms an integral part in the palliative care team's treatment plan for patients. Counselling skills to assess patients and an holistic approach to caring are key to the assessment process. The social worker will work directly with patients and families using individual, family, or group work techniques. Other colleagues may be involved when appropriate. The social worker's contribution helps to highlight that every patient is part of a social system which influences how they deal with their illness. Social system refers to the patient's cultural, religious, and social grouping and includes other factors such as age and sex. It also acknowledges the patient's role in their family and peer group. The patient is not just an individual with problems and symptoms, but a member of a family whose actions continually interact. Recognizing the patient as part of a family can be extremely helpful to the team since it provides the possibility of using the family's strength and resources, and reduces the team's need to be the 'sole saviours' (Smith 1990)

The diagnosis of a terminal illness can lead to personal confusion and isolation within a family. The social worker can work with a specific family helping to remove barriers by addressing conflicting feelings such as anger, guilt, sadness, and regret. Family members may have to take on unfamiliar roles, such as a wife taking on business responsibilities, or deal with the pain of losing a familiar role such as being a parent. Time and again, communication barriers appear because of pressure within the family to protect one another by not showing feelings. Joint interviews with a family by the social worker and nurse or doctor can be very helpful, especially if the family is large and there is considerable conflict to be understood. As a non-medical person, the social worker can act as a bridge between patients, families, and staff by helping the patient and the family to identify important questions and direct these to the appropriate staff members. With the greater pressure on hospice beds and the desire not to have increasing number of elderly cancer patients who are unsymptomatic blocking hospice beds, the social worker's input is invaluable to the team in coordinating nursing homes/community care support quickly.

Teenagers facing a serious illness such as leukaemia, or the unfortunate situation of a terminal illness, can be especially traumatic. In many units teenagers feel out of place—they are neither children nor adults. Fiercely trying to break out of the family as they approach adulthood and yet still desiring the caring and comfort, the teenager can bring complex problems to an often already difficult family situation as well as a busy ward. A social worker with specific skills in families, trained to work with teenagers, can be extremely useful. Such a specific role can be developed as part of the specialist social worker's wider remit where indicated. In the future the special needs of adolescents with cancer may be developed differently, but until then staff on busy acute wards will need specialist advice from someone. This role is part of the specialist social worker's job description on the palliative care team at the Western General Hospital NHS Trust, Edinburgh.

Responsibility for coordinating bereavement follow-up work may also be given to the social worker on the team. This may be organized for group work or individual contact depending on the size of the team. By listening, understanding, responding without being judgemental, and being able to tolerate unpleasant feelings, the social worker can prevent the bereaved from feeling overwhelmed and hopefully help them to move towards adjustment. Particular help is important for the younger children whose parent has died. Bereavement visits can encourage the family's questions about the death. These visits can be used to assess whether the person is at risk and requiring more specialist help or more in-depth support from local resources. All of this demonstrates that the family is still important, and provides an opportunity to say goodbye if contact is to end. The Gloucester Royal Infirmary Palliative Care Team have developed an extremely effective bereavement programme for children and their surviving parent (Stokes *et al.* 1997).

Besides having a clinical role, the social worker needs to be involved with the teaching activities of the team. Different team members seen teaching together, especially on issues of communication and families, can be an extremely effective way of showing individual professions the importance of interdisciplinary working. Having a social worker as a core member of the specialist palliative care team can lead to a more creative service for the patients and families, as well as providing for the individual and collective needs of the team. The social worker is often in a position to stand back from the medical and nursing aspects of patient care. They are able to monitor feelings within the team. The principles of counselling can be used within the team to precipitate sharing and caring, and this ensures that no individual is overwhelmed with responsibility.

Social workers employed by the local authority have certain statutory responsibilities not only to the elderly, sick, and handicapped, but also a wider mandate to children and the mentally ill. The social worker on the palliative care team may need to carry out responsibilities such as arranging emergency foster care for the baby of a dying single parent, or helping to assess a patient for compulsory care under the Mental Health Act as part of their work to social services even though a core member of the palliative care team.

Chaplain

Chaplains are widely available in the acute hospital setting to attend to the spiritual and religious needs of patients. Their role in the context of palliative care teams is often as a peripheral member rather than a core member. However, there are some chaplains who have been the voice behind the setting up of a palliative care team and thereby retained a substantial identity within the team. When this is the case he or she may be an important source of support and encouragement to the other team members, and may even be looked upon as a confidant. On occasions, the chaplain will facilitate examination and resolution of team conflict and stress, thereby improving the team dynamics.

Like all professionals, chaplains are human, and the degree of involvement with terminally ill patients varies. Some chaplains may limit their involvement to basic religious requirements such as administering the sacrament or reading the prayers for the dying. In the past less training was available at theological colleges on the needs of the dying and their families. Along with the hospice movement has come greater opportunity to look more deeply at spiritual and religious needs. Many chaplains enjoy opportunities for counselling patients and families, and participating in bereavement follow-up. Some chaplains will willingly sit with dying patients if the relatives are not available, and even go to the home of relatives to break bad news instead of the police or the dreaded telephone call.

The chaplain may also fulfil a consumer advocate role. It can be easier for a relative outsider to the medical and nursing professions to consider the patient and family perspective, thereby maintaining a more balanced, ethical approach. Chaplains who have dedicated time to a palliative care team may well be appreciated for being involved with ethical debates and problems. They are often willing to contribute actively to meetings, clinical situations, and written material if that is their interest.

The teaching role of the chaplain is a very important one, particularly if theological students visit the palliative care team. Often social workers and chaplains may work together. Chaplains with a more generic palliative care role, who are not part of the team, may teach and provide support on issues related to caring for the dying for medical, nursing, social work, and other students. This can be achieved by running support groups or small informal sessions where spiritual, ethical aspects of care and factors about coping with death and dying can be discussed.

It is very important for the palliative care team to build relationships with non-Christian spiritual advisers, particularly when minority groups are present within the district. Palliative care team members should take time to learn about the cultural and religious needs from these advisers and elders. The palliative care team can help to ensure that their comments are disseminated throughout the wards by means of informal teaching sessions, articles, and written documents, such as the *Care of the Dying* pamphlet published by the City and Hackney Health Authority, London.

Volunteers

Volunteers have been an integral part of the modern hospice movement. Many hospices would probably not survive were that not the case—certainly the quality of care would deteriorate. Within the acute hospital setting, volunteers do have a role but traditionally it is been confined to the running and organizing of hospital shops, transport, or a guide service helping people to find the various departments. A few hospital-based palliative care units train volunteers to be more actively involved in patient care (Brazil and Thomas 1995) but within the context of the peripatetic team, this can become complicated. The St Thomas's Hospital Terminal Care Support Team (Bates 1985) uses volunteers particularly for day care. At its inception, St Luke's Hospital Palliative Care Service in New York, used volunteers substantially (Kaplan and O'Connor 1989). Despite these examples, few hospital-based palliative care teams make use of volunteers.

This may be partly due to the rigorous organization that is required, such as provision of study days and training courses. This can be done if there is a volunteer coordinator. Even then, it is time consuming especially if the team only has two or three members. General volunteers appointed by hospitals have good support and training but volunteering to work with the care of the dying does require particular commitment and training.

Some of the occasions when volunteers have been used by hospital-based palliative care teams include the following:

- Providing transport for patients to clinics and day care facilities. The volunteer driver will frequently find themselves being party to patient's fears and anxieties as they travel to and from the clinic. This information may help the team to improve their understanding of the patient. It is important to clarify hospital policies about the legal and insurance requirements for transporting patients in private vehicles.
- Secretarial help.
- Shopping
- Bereavement follow-up when the volunteer has a background that qualifies them to be involved in this way.
- Sitting with patients whose families are unable to visit because they are too far away.
- Sitting with patients at night. This can take place at home and in the hospital. Patients without family, or whose family cannot visit, can be greatly comforted. The anxiety and guilt that the nursing staff feel about not being able to sit with dying patients will also be relieved.
- Visiting patients. The ability of some people to befriend patients who are socially isolated will also contribute to better patient care and lower stress levels. Patients may well share some problems that they would not otherwise be able to. It is important to recognize that some patients wish to retain a life-long reclusive tendency and will resent the intrusion of lay persons as much as health professionals.

Recruiting team members

When appointing additional team members to an emerging team, it is vital to consider the skills already present in the team as well as the candidates suitability for the job. If a team leader's interest and skills lie in symptom control or family work then appointing someone with audit, research, or computer skills is much more likely to complement and expand the service. Mount (1980) emphasizes the importance of not trying to 'sell' the post. The stress of working on a palliative care team must not be underplayed or covered up. There is considerable uncertainty about the best way of appointing new recruits and appointing into a small, highly motivated team is not an easy job.

A palliative care manual (Mount 1980) detailing how a palliative care service was set up in Montreal, Canada, states that within six months of the unit opening, serious errors had been recognized in the selection of four of their key leadership personnel. Apparently all the candidates were chosen for their exceptional standard as nurses; however, this does not necessarily equate with exceptional 'leadership' qualities. The committee investigating the situation looked to see if there were any common factors between the appointments—not looking at personality types but actual issues around the hiring contract. In each case there were three concurring themes:

- Paucity of applicants for the job—palliative care was quite a new field in Canada in the early 1980s and so people with this expertise were limited.
- Incomplete analysis of the job requirements and the applicants capabilities.
- A sense of urgency to fill the position.

This example highlights issues which are also important for staff selection to a palliative care team. The right criteria for selection must be assessed before considering whether or not the right selection method is being used. Too often the haphazard nature of selection is realised after a person is in post.

The formal interview is repeatedly seen as one of the most difficult ways of assessing a candidate and a large body of research going back to the early part of this century shows that selection through interviewing *alone* is useless (Cook 1988). However, it is a brave person who will scrap the interview altogether. The interview is often seen as the selecting process 'all in one' rather than the final piecing together of what is quite a complex jigsaw puzzle. Research has shown (Plumbley 1991) that there are six basic faults that interviewers face, the majority of which can be attributed to lack of appropriate preparation. One of the important things to consider is the selection of the interview panel. One of the advantages of panel interviewing is that there is less danger of nepotism (Hyett 1984). More than one interviewer gives more time to reflect during the interview, making it easier to record relevant aspects. There is always the danger of a dominant personality on the panel swaying the final choice.

'Group selection' has been used in appointing various different team members to several palliative care teams. It can be used in various ways, either formally or informally. Within the formal setting all the candidates would meet together with some of the members of the team and a subject chosen for the group to discuss. A more informal way would be for other members of the palliative care team to join the candidates for lunch. This method can provide additional information about social, interaction, and attitudinal skills within small groups. Generally 'group selection' is done alongside panel interviewing.

Presentation skills may need to be assessed, especially when selecting nurse specialists or medical personnel to the team. Teaching is increasingly an integral part of the work of a palliative care team. The candidate will be asked to perform a small presentation, generally lasting only 8–10 minutes, on an aspect relevant to the job in question. Aspects to notice include how well researched the presentation is, the content, and the ability to keep to time. If the presentation is done first, then often the candidate will relax for the panel interview.

An examination of past work habits should seek to establish whether the candidate can set and achieve realistic goals (LaGrand 1980). Past education and training should routinely be scrutinized. Breadth of experience is one of the most important factors that a member can bring to a palliative care team. A recent bereavement or other significant stress may render the candidate unsuitable, albeit temporarily. Because the work is often emotionally exhausting, a candidate's general physical health must be good. Discussion with previous employers (not necessarily just the most recent) should evaluate character traits such as stability, ability to relate well, perseverance and leadership ability. Flippancy, poor self-control, dependence, inability to accept responsibility, and show-off tendencies will seriously detract from a person's ability to perform in a supportive, advisory role. Conversely, people with the strong sense of self, necessary to withstand the stresses of this field, may be less able to function in a team.

It is important to understand why the candidate is applying for the post. Mary Vachon (1978, 1987) has elucidated the motives of people working in terminal care. Some people drift into applying for the job because of the convenience of hours or such like; others seek to master the difficulties of illness and dying, or master colleagues by becoming an adviser. A sense of 'calling' may imply a stable philosophy and strong background support but can lead to a crusading approach that overpowers patient, family, and staff. Another double-edged motive is the desire to disprove past failures and demonstrate skills which the candidate perceives have been suppressed in previous jobs. The credentials of any person employed must evoke respect from other nursing and medical staff.

The final decision about who is appointed should be made on the basis of which applicant has the closest match between capabilities, personality characteristics, and idiosyncrasies; and the job requirements. Some degree of compromise will be inevitable. It is vital that the selection committee do not feel compelled to appoint if the degree of mismatch is too great. The apparent needs of the terminally ill and the ready availability of charity money to start a service will conspire to generate a sense of urgency. This urgency must be resisted if a suitable candidate is not forthcoming. Hasty, stop-gap appointments can seriously jeopardize the mental and physical well-being of the person appointed, quite apart from the quality and credibility of the service.

The appointment of team members is merely a prelude to the next difficult phase. The individuals must begin providing a service, and weld themselves into a team. The next chapters examine how the team members interact with patients, families, other staff, and with each other.

4

Achieving change without power

Thirty years have passed since the founding of the modern hospice movement. Health professionals and the lay public are more aware of the importance of palliative care. Government planning for health care will often explicitly include care for the dying. Palliative medicine has now realized specialty status in many countries. In the UK and Australasia, the specialty is affiliated to the respective College of Physicians. The body of knowledge about palliative care continues to expand rapidly. Several academic departments have been created. Articles about this field now regularly appear in top-rated journals such as the *British Medical Journal* and the *Lancet*, as well as in the specialist journals pertaining to palliative care. It is not uncommon for national and international meetings about cancer treatments to include some mention of palliative care. Medical and nursing students rarely graduate without having heard of the specialty, even if the depth of teaching about pain control, breaking bad news, and other issues is still inadequate.

The higher profile of palliative care is encouraging more health care professionals and policy-makers to recognize the value of hospital-based palliative care teams. In the UK, the Department of Health realizes that most people die in acute hospitals. There is a deeply felt concern to ensure that these people have access to high standards of terminal care. The NHS Executive have required that purchasers of health care must have clear plans for developing palliative care, alongside cancer services generally. Guidance on this process from the National Council of Hospice and Specialist Palliative Care Services has mentioned palliative care teams. The ready availability of pump-priming money from Macmillan Cancer Relief has helped to overcome the financial barriers for setting up teams. All of these factors will encourage the growing numbers of hospital-based palliative care teams.

Although palliative care is more widely understood and accepted, this does not mean that a new hospital palliative care team will be universally welcomed. The manager who champions the new team will often be encouraged by a small group of enthusiastic senior medical and nursing staff. However, many clinical staff will be antipathetic, occasionally even hostile. This atmosphere is made more daunting for new teams by their own realization of the levels of unmet need in patients and families. There will also be the pressure to demonstrate the cost-effectiveness of the team. It is difficult enough for other services to meet these demands when they have direct control over the care of patients. Hospital palliative care teams have to achieve change without having any power. They must work alongside other staff who are responsible for delivering care, thereby achieving the results by which the team will be judged.

This chapter addresses the issue of achieving change without power and direct authority. Parallels will be drawn between palliative care teams and modern organizations which have to earn the loyalty of employees, rather than expect it by right. The value of systems thinking will be highlighted as a framework by which a palliative care team, new or established, should approach the issue of change within an organization. The chapter will conclude by reviewing the strategies which can be used to influence and promote change in the absence of authority.

Managing without power in the business world

Although the challenges of improving palliative care are specific to palliative care teams, the problems of managing change without authority are not unique. More generally, social forces are undermining the traditional respect for formal authority. Relationships between teachers and students are more relaxed in schools. Television and other media encourage self-reliance and emphasize individual rights. As people have become better educated, they have developed greater distrust of systems. These factors are changing the hierarchical bureaucratic style of business management. Political initiatives such as deregulation mean that previous ways of working cannot be taken for granted. Economic forces are also compounding the sense of rapid change. These changes demand greater flexibility, particularly as companies compete in the global marketplace. With the passing of 'jobs for life', workers are looking for personal challenges which can further their career prospects.

As more businesses adopt flatter, non-hierarchical structures, the usual directive management approach is becoming outmoded. The task of facilitating rather than demanding change has grown in importance. Psychologists and management consultants have been developing new strategies in light of these challenges. These strategies provide valuable insights and guidance for palliative care teams. The next sections deal with the concepts of systems thinking and personal mastery, as popularized by Senge (1990). Following this, there is a review of the various influence processes which have been identified.

Systems thinking

The task of setting up a palliative care team can be very daunting. Acute hospitals are large organizations. Terminally ill patients will be cared for in many different wards, alongside patients with the full range of other medical and surgical conditions. The wards will all be different, with staff having different skills and needs. Where do you start? How can you possibly fulfil the expectations of the managers and the funders of the team? The temptation is to simplify the task, adopting a uniform approach which tries to cover all of the wards. Inevitably, this leads to setbacks and frustrations that can overwhelm the initial enthusiasm.

Systems thinking is a body of knowledge and tools which can guide you in planning the process of change. It is based on the premise that organizations such as hospitals are systems, in which complex interrelated actions are bound together. The relationships between individuals, wards, and departments will seem complicated when seen in isolation. Systems thinking looks at the whole, seeking to identify patterns which underlie these complex situations. These patterns will often conform to systems archetypes, which are models of recurrent behaviour patterns. Senge (1990) has reviewed several of these models

There is one particular systems archetype which is very relevant to the situation faced by a palliative care team. It is known as 'limits to growth'. This paradigm begins by describing the effects of any process which is put in place to achieve growth. If the process is successful, then a positive feedback loop will develop. Success will breed further success in a reinforcing upward spiral. For example, a palliative care team which achieves spectacular early results might generate confidence in referring doctors. This would lead to further clinical success thereby reinforcing the desire of other doctors to refer to the team. However, the 'limits to growth' model also has a balancing loop which operates in the opposite direction. A balancing loop has the effect of maintaining stability. Thus, in most systems which are exposed to change, the initial reaction is to prevent this change from upsetting the *status quo*. This model explains why most teams will initially experience a cautious, occasionally antagonistic response. It also explains why little progress will be seen, especially on wards where key staff such as consultants are suspicious of the service.

The 'limits to growth' archetype contains other important insights. The consequences of a balancing loop which opposes a reinforcing growth loop is captured in the quote 'the harder you push the system, the harder it will push you back' (Senge 1990). Most new palliative care teams feel under pressure to make an early impact and achieve noticeable change. The natural instinct is to try to push 'the system'. This is more likely when a team member becomes frustrated and impatient for change. A difficult case, such as a consultant refusing to action advice about a distressing symptom, will then trigger an assertive response. Unfortunately, this is more likely to produce the opposite reaction, a hardening of the consultant's attitude and a reluctance to refer future patients.

There is a more effective way to produce change. Rather than push for growth, it is better to look for high-leverage opportunities which reduce the resistance to change. For example, a ward team may be loath to refer new patients. The consultant may even have openly questioned the value of creating the team. However, after the team has been in operation for a while, the consultant might allow a referral to be made. The patient will usually be very 'difficult' in some way: 'blocking' a bed for too long, making 'unreasonable' demands , a 'problem' family which is disrupting the ward. By waiting until this type of opportunity arises and then spending a lot of effort sorting out the situation, you will gain a lot more credibility and open up more chances for the team to be involved in the future.

'Limits to growth' also predicts the effects of success on the team as it becomes more widely accepted. When the team starts, referrals will be slow in coming. Gradually, the workload of the team will increase. As the impact of the team grows, more staff will want to refer patients earlier in the course of the illness. Eventually, the workload will exceed the capacity of the palliative care team. Then, delays will occur before new referrals are seen. If the team is too busy, patients will not be seen as often as they would have been when the team started. Potentially, the quality of the service will suffer, which might decrease the number of referrals. In practice, ward staff do not notice a significant difference but the palliative care team comes under greater stress. It always takes a long time to fund, recruit, and train new team members. Therefore, when referrals start to increase, this should signal the need for advance planning rather than just signal time for celebration and self-congratulation.

Another important insight which is derived from systems archetypes is the significance of delays between actions and their consequences. The results of actions, such as setting up a palliative care team, are rarely apparent immediately. The relevance of this insight was illustrated in the previous example about planning ahead when referrals start to increase. The most difficult example for team members to cope with is the long delay in seeing improvements in patient and family care. Small gains will be made on individual wards as the palliative care team becomes more involved. However, these gains can be easily undermined when there is a change of junior medical staff. Even more distressing are the examples where ward staff do not take advice, leaving patients to suffer unnecessarily. Even when a team has been operating for several years, these examples still arise. Team members need to develop methods for dealing with the psychological effects of these delays. One method is the discipline of personal mastery.

Personal mastery

Personal mastery is one of the five disciplines described by Senge (1990). Along with systems thinking, it is used to facilitate 'learning' organizations which are able to learn from the past and adapt flexibly to the future. The principles of personal mastery are also useful for palliative care teams. Personal mastery is not about conquering or dominating situations or people. This would be the complete antithesis of the advisory role. Instead, personal mastery involves the constant clarification and deepening of your personal vision. You need to have a compelling view of how excellent palliative care could be delivered in the acute hospital environment. What benefits would accrue to the patients, the families, and the staff? It is important to develop a shared vision across the team but vision is also about continually clarifying what is important to you, aligning your ultimate intrinsic desires with the broader vision. It should generate commitment, involvement, and desire for change. While your vision may be usefully informed by having worked in a hospice, there are greater challenges in the hospital environment. The essence of palliative care is to help patients and families maximize their sense of control and achievement in the face of progressive loss. Achieving this in the hospital environment is not just at the heart of palliative care, it is at the heart of all medicine.

At the same time as you develop a vision for the future, you need to maintain a clear objective understanding of reality. People who are faced with seemingly unattainable goals will either distort reality (perceive things as better than they really are) or they weaken the vision. The gap between vision and reality often generates emotional tensions, such as frustration, anger, anxiety, and eventually despair. Personal mastery encourages you to use the gap as a creative tension. You need to be disciplined about developing patience, channelling the potential negative energies into finding and exploiting the opportunities for moving toward the vision.

Understanding the process of influence

There are many ways in which power is exercized within organizations. Bragg (1996) described seven 'power levers' which are used to achieve change:

1. Resources: control over the availability of scarce resources.
2. Information: may also be used as a means of control and influence. This includes technical information as well as knowledge about important relationships and networks
3. Expertise: knowledge about highly specialized subjects
4. Connections with outside organizations and people. These may include professional and personal links.
5. Coercion: use of a punishment-centred approach.
6. Position within the hierarchical power structure will give the individual power to allocate, make decisions, hire and fire, etc.
7. Personal power such as charisma and personality. Some people can exercise considerable influence with their personal charisma but this tends not to be long-lasting.

Palliative care teams do not have many of these options available to them. They are rarely in a position to use coercion or power. Expertise is the most powerful lever, particularly in light of the distress which other staff experience when caring for the terminally ill. This re-emphasizes the value of appointing well-trained team members. There may be some control over the availability of resources. Many teams control the availability of syringe drivers or other pumps which are used to infuse medications such as morphine when patients are no longer able to swallow. Technical knowledge is usually limited to the few technical issues specific to palliative care. The knowledge which teams acquire by moving about the hospital can be very helpful. You can build up strong relationships and networks across departments and disciplines. This can be exploited on behalf of ward staff, for example by expediting a very important investigation.

The principles of influence

There are other ways in which palliative care teams can effect change. Before considering these in detail, it is helpful to review what determines whether people respond to influence. Bragg (1996) identified six principles of influence:

1. Historical commitments and consistency. People have an overwhelming desire to act in ways that reinforce and justify their past decisions and actions. This principle will count against you if you are trying to change bad practices. Staff will resist acknowledging that previous care has been poor. However, you can use this principle to reinforce examples of good practice.
2. Contrast. Although the present is often used to ratify the past, the contrast between what is happening and what is possible can occasionally unlock the desire for change.
3. Scarcity. If something is rarely available, it will often become more desirable. This happened to a palliative care team which attempted a randomized study of their service. Some wards were randomly assigned to receive visits from the team. The trial folded because the other wards transferred patients to the wards in the experimental arm (Davies, personal communication).
4. Social proof: the reliance that people place on the opinions and behaviours of others. Decisions and actions are then based on the desire to fit in with what everyone is doing. This principle will increasingly act in favour of effective palliative care teams. Staff will share experiences about the team between the wards and departments, creating an atmosphere in which referral to the team is the expected norm.
5. Liking and ingratiation. People are more likely to be influenced by someone with whom they feel comfortable. Factors such as physical attractiveness, similar social status, compliments, and flattery will all have a positive influence. Palliative care teams often use these factors,

for example in deciding to use a doctor to speak with another consultant.

6. Emotion. Although health professionals like to believe that decisions are made objectively, emotions exert just as much influence as intellect. You can influence the behaviour of others by the way you express your emotions. It is important to learn how best to use your emotions in the advisory role.

Tactics for influencing change

Yukl and Falbe (1990) carried out a study of the ways in which influence is exercized in business. They found that a wide range of tactics were used. Different tactics were used according to whether the person was trying to influence a superior, a peer, or a subordinate:

1. Pressure tactics entailing the use of demands, threats, and intimidation. These tactics are rarely if ever appropriate in the advisory role.
2. Upward appeals are used to influence subordinates. In an effort to persuade staff of the importance of a particular initiative, the support of senior managers is used to emphasize the need for change. This approach is also rarely used by palliative care teams. Occasionally, a senior hospital manager has required a team to work with a particular ward, for example when there have been complaints from relatives about the care on the ward. The team may need to use an upward appeal to begin the process of change. However, a mandate from management is unlikely to make the ward staff more receptive to the advice of the team.
3. Rational appeals involve the use of logical arguments and facts to persuade others. This is often needed to give doctors and nurses more confidence when you advise the use of new or unfamiliar treatments.
4. Exchange tactics are based on the principle of reciprocity: if you do something for me, I will do something for you. This is usually not made explicit. However, team members will sometimes accept requests for teaching from a doctor who does not normally use the team in the hope that this will facilitate relationships in the future.
5. Coalition tactics rely on building up a group of people who will support your efforts. In general, it is unwise to be too closely aligned to particular wards or departments in the hospital. However, there is a tendency for a group of supportive individuals to develop over time.

The group will not exist as a specific entity but will exert influence on your behalf, particularly with senior management.

6. Ingratiation tactics operate by getting the person into a good mood or thinking positively. The term 'ingratiation' has a negative connotation. It suggests that you have to grovel or fawn to get results. This would never work with health professionals. In fact, it would be counter-productive. However, the appropriate use of praise, humour, and similar approaches is very important for palliative care teams.

7. Inspirational appeals make use of emotional petitions to arouse enthusiasm. This has some value when you are teaching students. However, there are few opportunities for inspirational appeals in the clinical setting. The effects of inspirational appeals tend to be short-lived.

8. Consultation tactics involve staff in the process of making a decision or planning how to implement change. Consultation tactics are becoming more widely used in business because they promote a greater sense of ownership in the change process. This can also be useful in the clinical setting. One example is to get groups of staff together to develop protocols for palliative care, such as the breaking of bad news or the use of morphine. The protocols will have limited influence outside the group but the participants will be better informed. The team will develop better relationships with the staff as well.

How to become influential in the advisory role

The first step to becoming more influential is to know yourself and your colleagues on the team (see chapter 6). Your beliefs, values, and assumptions will all have an effect on the way you interact with others. You need to be aware of your weaknesses, for example the tendency to get angry when faced with 'incompetence'. Strong negative emotions need to be controlled if you are supporting other staff. When you are faced with a difficult clinical situation, you should try to take the time to thoroughly analyse the circumstances. Who are the crucial staff members? What are their behaviours, values, attitudes, and ideas? Your evaluation should include verbal and non-verbal cues, organizational factors, and any personal issues. Systems thinking will help you to understand the relationship between the hidden systems of hospital and the influences on the ward team. As you appraise the situation, you should be deciding on the most appropriate strategy and tactics. A variety of influence tactics are usually needed, which match the objectives and audience. In general, soft influence tactics are better than confrontational or domineering tactics.

Bragg (1996) advises a systematic approach to developing your influence skills. You must become familiar with the principles and tactics of influence. The references in this chapter contain more information. It is then important to practice using influence. Feedback from team members should be used to refine the skills. With time, you will find that the skills get integrated into your clinical repertoire, becoming second nature to you. This will give you more confidence for dealing with high-pressure situations where time is short and emotions are running high.

Summary

Palliative care teams have a difficult role in acute hospitals. The team must improve the care of terminally ill patients by giving advice and support. Their influence is indirect and is not based on traditional power structures. This situation is analogous to the management issues facing modern companies. Team members need to see the process of change as a slow gradual one, punctuated by frustrations and delays. The tension between this reality and your vision for palliative care will be helped by the discipline of personal mastery. You should become familiar with the principles and tactics of influence. The team will function more effectively if the team members practice these strategies together.

5

The ethical basis for making decisions

Decisions about care at the end of life are very difficult. It is often distressing looking after terminally ill patients and their families. This makes decisions about witholding or withdrawing life-prolonging treatment even more emotive. One only has to consider the number of people involved in making treatment decisions—the patient, the family, the nurses, and the doctors—to realize that the potential for conflict is enormous. Into this situation comes the hospital-based palliative care team, a 'problem solving, decision-making mechanism' (Beckhard 1974) which can only advise. It is essential for team members to have a sound understanding of the ethical basis for making decisions. Otherwise, they will simply be adding yet another opinion to the conflict.

When difficult ethical issues arise, team members should take time to discuss the issues with each other before going back to the referring team. There are usually several factors which must be taken into account, and sometimes it is helpful to clarify one's thoughts with other members of the palliative care team first. There may be no 'right answer' but arguing from a set of basic ethical principles helps to organize one's thoughts more rationally.

This chapter briefly outlines the basis of ethical principles. It includes ideas on exploring what the patient understands about future treatment and how to present treatment options. Some of the major ethical dilemmas within the context of hospital palliative care are discussed including euthanasia and living wills.

Basic ethical principles

Current medical ethics emphasize that patient choice is central to the decision-making process (Beauchamp and Childress 1983). Patients are autonomous individuals capable of choosing their treatment and care. Making decisions for a patient, without their consent, is only ethically justified when they are not capable of understanding or making decisions themselves. One cannot label patients as incompetent just because they appear uncooperative. However, patients who are confused, psychotic, demented, or comatose when dying may be unable to comprehend or decide. Severely depressed patients may also have difficulty making decisions. Any wishes expressed by patients before they become incompetent must be taken into account.

Team members need to be well versed in the four ethical principles:

- autonomy
- beneficence (doing good)
- non-maleficence (doing no harm)
- justice

in order to understand some of the basic issues in decision-making.

Autonomy is generally applied to the patient's situation but there is an argument that doctors have a degree of professional autonomy regarding treatments. However, there is no place for strong paternalism, which threatens autonomy. For example, an anti-cancer treatment with minimal effectiveness may be witheld by the doctor who overemphasizes the 'do no harm' principle, which usurps the right of the patient who wants the treatment because it will 'do good'. Using the four ethical principles enables greater clarity in complex situations especially when the various arguments are emotionally charged. Even when a patient is fully informed about current illness and the options, there are many factors and situations that cause uncertainty about the 'right thing' to do.

Gillon (1994) takes these four principles one step further by adding 'attention to scope'. Some of the moral issues that arise in health care come from differing cultural, philosophical, political, and religious backgrounds. Seeing the dilemma within the context of these backgrounds is an important approach and makes it easier to apply the ethical principles within the specific clinical situation.

In an approach focused on the ethics of palliative care, Jeffrey (1993) has developed an ethical model with four facets (see Table 5.1):

- respect for autonomy
- a caring partnership
- a shared culture
- care for the carers.

This is an interesting example of a model designed within the framework

Table 5.1   Model for the ethics of palliative care (Jeffrey 1993)

Respect for autonomy	Avoiding 'strong' paternalism which threatens autonomy
	Adopting a broad approach to autonomy which permits 'weak' paternalism
	Sharing truthful information about diagnosis, treatment, and prognosis with the patient, in a sensitive manner
	Presenting the patient with choices
	Seeking the patient's free, informed, and understood consent
A caring partnership	A partnership between doctors, other health care professionals and the patient based on trust and an open honest approach
	A holistic approach to care
	A commitment to teamwork, a partnership between health carers
	Acknowledging uncertainty and vulnerability
	Listening to the patient
	Avoiding distancing, sharing emotional involvement and compassion with the patient and his or her family
A shared culture	Promoting the acceptance of death
	Resolving unfinished business
	Demystifying cancer and death
	Acknowledging the value of life and rejecting active euthanasia
	Accepting that 'letting die' may be permissible in some circumstances
	Making an appropriate transition between a curative and a palliative approach to care, with the patient's consent and comprehension
	Taking account of the patient's view on the quality of his or her life
Care for the carers	Supporting the patient's family
	Supporting doctors and nurses and other health care professionals
	Recognizing and avoiding burnout

of a definite culture. It was designed for hospice but much of it can be applied to the hospital-based palliative care team.

Gathering information from the patient

When asked to see a patient, one must define what the problems are, and who has which problem. Team members will soon learn that hospital staff may present problems such as pain when it is actually the staff who are having difficulty coping with the patient.

The first task is to find out what the patient perceives to be the problems. Begin with open-ended questions such as 'how is it affecting you?' When the patient has described his needs, direct questions may be used to check specific issues or details. You should try not to put words in the patient's mouth. If a patient wants to ignore or deny distress from symptoms then this must be respected. It demonstrates a commitment to the patient's wishes and will allow him to maintain a sense of control. It also saves the team and the patient from the stress of dealing with issues that are not currently important to the patient.

Once you have identified the patient's problems then you can check what the patient wants and begin devising potential solutions. Inevitably there will be some issues that cannot be resolved, for example the wish to be cured. Most patients comprehend this fact, even if they have not been explicitly told. However, some patients focus on this issue as their main problem. Rather than confront the patient's perception, it may be more helpful to talk sensitively about the fears of not being cured. This can be followed by opportunities to help the patient take more control of the weeks and months ahead.

Finding out what the patient wants is vital, but the principle of comparative justice recognizes that the choice of the patient is not absolute. Nonetheless it is difficult to ignore a patient's insistence for further chemotherapy which is unlikely to help and may be life-threatening. Time spent trying to understand why the patient is so insistent on further chemotherapy can be a real support for the oncology team involved. They may also be very ambivalent about giving further treatment when time is spent understanding the issues; patients and their families feel more reassured that decisions have been made with due consideration of their own interests. Presenting the options and the final decision is then often less traumatic.

Presenting options to patients

As problems are defined, possible solutions can be devised. These strategies should be presented to the patient. There should be opportunities for patients and family to ask questions about potential risks and benefits, and alternative treatments. Patients should also have time to deliberate, if they want. The team should endeavour to support the patient's choice, but should remember that patients may change their views with time.

Sometimes patients find it difficult to participate in discussions about strategies for their needs because they fear that the doctors may take umbrage. It is little wonder, when you read the St Bartholomew's Hospital rules published circa 1900. Rule 7 stated that 'every patient must strictly obey the Directions of the Physician or Surgeon under whose care he or she may be placed'. Compliance was ensured by the concluding rule; 'any patient acting contrary to the foregoing Rules will be reported by the Sister of the Ward to the Steward or Matron, and by them to the Treasurer: such Patient will be admonished or discharged'. It is also important to recognize that, while a patient may initially agree to a particular treatment, later non-compliance should be recognized as a choice, rather than the patient being regarded as 'unreasonable' or 'ungrateful'. Failure to cooperate is one of the few tactics that patients have for maintaining control.

Maintaining the precedence of informed patient choice can be very difficult, particularly if the team members have a palliative care philosophy of minimizing active treatment. In the hospital situation the patient should not become a battle field between the 'care oriented' team member and the 'cure oriented' hospital teams. Patients may well accept a considerable degree of risk from treatments which hold minimal chances of benefit.

In practice, it may be extremely difficult to present alternatives to the patient, particularly when the primary team is not willing or likely to fulfil the patient's choice. In some circumstances, a patient will be referred because he or she wants more treatment than the primary team are prepared to give. The expectation of the primary team will be that the team member will persuade the patient to accept their decision. You must never lose sight of these expectations but, for the patient's sake, try to look beyond them. As the palliative care team becomes more established, and especially when there is a medical presence on the team, debates about the relative merits of treatment become easier to discuss with referring consultants and their teams.

Balancing patient wishes with family and staff

It is always important to speak to both the patient's relatives *and* the staff as well as the patient, particularly when ethical dilemmas have precipitated the referral. Valuable information can be obtained about symptoms or psychosocial difficulties, and it may be possible to find out about past experiences of cancer which are dictating what the patient presents or how they interpret information (Billings 1985). This additional information should not override the patient's perceptions, but it may subsequently facilitate the expression of fears about symptoms or treatment.

Patients know best how their body is feeling, especially as they approach death. However, many health care professionals make decisions based on test results alongside the clinical situation without really taking the time to understand how the patient is feeling. Members of the palliative care team have a vital role to play in listening to what the different 'parties' are saying.

Some patients have a premonition of death a week or so before they die. If they have courage enough, and if they are given the opportunity, they may talk about this. Requests to 'go home to die' need to be taken seriously, however inconvenient they may be on a Friday morning. Such a request is often too complicated for ward staff to organize on their own. The palliative care team needs to be willing to help coordinate the arrangements, making sure that the necessary nursing and medical help are alerted so that the discharge home does not end up as a disaster. The needs of the family are important. Sometimes their needs conflict with those of the patient, for example if they will have to care for the patient at home but they do not want to. Generally, patients and families requesting such a decision know what they are asking for and have the inner resources to cope with emergencies as long as routine help is available.

Occasionally members of the palliative care team have to stand by a carefully thought through decision that they have made in the best interest of patient and family, despite it being contrary to a particular request. Some decisions are proved right, others sadly backfire. It is important to learn from these successes and failures. However, it is also important to remember that if in doubt a patient *and* family's considered request and decision is difficult to refute.

Ethical dilemmas in palliative care

Latimer (1991), in referring to the four ethical principles and their role in palliative care ethics, states that the autonomous patient's wishes should take precedence wherever possible. Treatment decisions should be made jointly by the patient and physician. If this guidance could be followed by all concerned then many of the ethical dilemmas discussed below would not be such big issues. Unfortunately, because of circumstances and human failure, situations are often not quite so straightforward.

'Active' versus 'palliative' treatments

'Active' treatments are anti-cancer therapies such as surgery, radiotherapy, and chemotherapy. 'Palliative' treatments are therapies such as analgesics, anti-emetics, etc. which relieve symptoms but do not affect the underlying cancer.

Debating the merits of 'active' versus 'palliative' treatments in someone with advanced, incurable cancer can be taxing, especially in the context of an oncology ward that is used to using fourth- and fifth-line chemotherapy. In such situations its best not only to consider each patient and family case individually, but also to apply the four main ethical arguments (see above). In effect, decisions re 'active' versus 'palliative' treatment is probably more explicitly described as end-of-life decision-making. This can help to focus some of the conversations more appropriately.

When there are unambiguous decisions from medical experts that aggressive treatment for metastatic disease is unlikely to benefit the patient, then further discussion about other care options is usually more clear cut. In practice, however, the clinical setting is always influenced by differing personalities, emotional involvement of patients and their families, and staff. What seems clear cut in the theoretical analysis of decision-making is often fraught with anguish when you are face to face with patient and family. How decisions are accepted by patients and their families is often influenced by length of illness, their satisfaction with care prior to diagnosis and during illness, their trust of the medical and nursing staff, support, and their previous knowledge and understanding of disease and specific treatments (Latimer 1991).

One of the most difficult situations in end-of-life decision-making involves the young oncology patient who has had a previous unexpected, dramatic response to chemotherapy. Despite progression of disease there is often a desire to find similar chemotherapy to give the same response. Clearly there is a danger in losing sight of the situation because of the heightened emotional involvement in the 'battle' against cancer. In situations like this, the amount of input from the palliative care team will depend on how comfortable those making such difficult decisions are with themselves, and with the members of the palliative care team present. There will be times when it appears very appropriate for the palliative care team to be fully involved. Other times, you will sense that to be involved will just muddle an already complex situation. To remain quiet but present at ward rounds (especially if the team does not have a consultant/doctor full-time) can be the wise choice. Often, the earlier you have been involved in the recurrence scenario with the patient and family and the treatment team, the easier it is to be party to the 'end-of-life decision-making' process. However, it is impossible to be so fully involved with *all* patients in a busy cancer centre.

Sometimes team members advocate life-prolonging treatments in situations where an important event is being anticipated, such as a daugher or son's wedding. Such decisions can only be successfully made when complete and considered discussion has been made with all concerned, including patient and family, general practitioner, hospital doctors, and nurses. This is best done as a planned meeting rather than a hasty decision made during an unplanned discussion. In such a situation it is important that the consultant or senior doctor in charge of the patient is helped to orchestrate the discussions with the patient and family. This can be time consuming but very gratifying, especially when life is prolonged enough to make the intervention worthwhile without it then becoming a burden. It can be useful to attempt to see the 'way out' of a life-prolonging procedure or treatment, or how life might naturally come to an end before embarking on it. Throughout the process, the team should remain aware of the potential for the patient's condition to deteriorate before the event occurs.

Collusion with relatives

Collusion occurs when health professionals and family agree not to tell the patient about his diagnosis. Understanding and resolving collusion between patient and relatives can be both time consuming and complex. Collusion at its worst can be called 'deceit', but this is rarely how relatives and families understand such a situation. More often than not, the underlying motive is the desire to shield the patient from the horror of knowing the full situation. This reaction is a worthy one, but unfortunately it can never be sustained unless the patient wants this. In the end, the dying person's own body will reveal the inevitable truth. This is brilliantly portrayed in Tolstoy's novel *The Death of Ivan Illyich*.

Collusion is often one situation that the hospital-based palliative care team will be asked to help unravel because of the distress felt by the ward nurses, as well as the time involved working with the patient and the family. It is within the hospital setting that collusion often starts. We have all known the various scenarios. For example, anxious relatives wait for the surgeon to appear from the operating theatre in order to hear the outcome of the operation; before the surgeon realizes, he or she has consented to the relatives' request not to inform the patient of the seriousness of the condition.

It is important never to 'blame' either party but to work out a strategy that will help to bring about a resolution and more open communication. Generally the referral is often requested because the patient has started to ask questions that the doctors and nurses find difficult because of the relatives' strict instructions not to inform. It will depend on the demands from the family as to whether the team member sees the patient first or the family. Generally it is best, whatever the demands, to see the patient first (as one would with any other referral) and then meet the family. It may be that because of the ongoing collusion, no one to date has sat and talked in any depth with the patient. If this is the case then the patient may have insight into the situation facing them because of the way people have been reacting. It often takes a good deal of concentration, effort, and skill to conduct such an interview but it can be extremely rewarding.

When seeing the patient it is important to remember to make a point of saying that you would like to meet the family. Just as you have seen the patient alone and had time to talk through some of his or her difficulties, it is important that the family have the opportunity of talking about what is worrying them. In this way it gives you permission to spend time with the family legitimately.

Very occasionally it might be right to meet the family first to hear their reasons for not wanting the patient to be told. However, you then run the danger of being drawn into the collusion. Often the team member's attitude and understanding of the situation will give the relatives confidence to realize that an already difficult situation will not be made worse. It is important for relatives to come to trust the skill of the team member.

The family's main worries often revolve around:

- not wanting to be found out that they have known all along
- fear that they won't be able to handle their own emotions when the patient is told
- fear that the patient won't be able to cope
- fear that the patient might give up because that is what has happened previously
- fear that bad news might be delivered in a harsh way.

If you can get the family to open up they are often exhausted by having to 'cover their tracks' in the collusion.

Just occasionally the family is right and the patient should not be told. However, this is very rare. Sometimes a patient gives a clue by admitting 'it's best if you talk to the wife' when asked if he would like to know all the results of the various tests.

In some situations, communication between the patient and family has been poor for many years. Unravelling such long-term difficulties may not be possible. Working with whatever the patient and family can share and deal with is important, but sometimes it is too late to make any impact of lasting value. Such situations are less than ideal and may require long-term follow up during the bereavement phase. However, it is worth remembering that the patient and the family will have different expectations about resolving their 'normal' pattern of behaviour.

Patients who decline treatment

In the current climate of financial constraint in health care, it might be assumed that a patient declining expensive anti-cancer treatment would be a source of relief. However, this is often not the case, because the medical staff will have been made to feel powerless to help the patients. The palliative care team may be asked to advise in this situation. However, this can be fraught with difficulties especially if the medical team are still hoping that the patient will agree to treatment. The medical team may want the palliative care team to change the patient's mind.

Decisions about treatment for patients are never just confined to the patient and medical team. Often the family 'side' with the medical team because of their grief that the patient will die more quickly. The patient can be very isolated, and it needs the palliative care team to try to untangle the various emotional responses resulting from such a situation. Bits of the jigsaw need to be collected and pieced together. This is best done by speaking to all the various parties involved, often more than once: the patient and the family (on their own as well as together), the nursing and medical staff. It is then easier to start understanding the complexities of the situation. Often it may be necessary to ask a second member of the palliative care team to come and at least meet the patient in order to bring further clarity on the situation.

In other cases the patient may be depressed. Because of the low mood, the patient cannot face being 'put through' any more. It may be possible to come to a compromise and delay treatment decisions while the depression is treated. Alternatively, it may be that the patient really knows what he or she wants and is perfectly capable of making a rational decision. Then the palliative care team must act as an advocate on behalf of the patient, while enabling the family to cope with the various emotions generated by such a decision. Often families who have wanted further treatment might feel very angry towards the patient for denying treatment. It will be important to stress the role that 'symptom control' has within such a situation, and that the patient and family will not be isolated from help just because no further active treatment is being given.

These situations can really highlight the expertise of a palliative care team. The help given in unravelling such complex issues can often ensure further referrals to the team in the future.

Sometimes the patient will refuse treatments recommended by the palliative care team. The patient may have been referred because of a refusal to take pain-killers. If the patient is obviously in pain but still refuses analgesics despite talking to the team, then the team members can feel very distressed. They may feel that they are failing and therefore redouble their persuasive efforts. However, this only alienates the patient. It is more helpful to support the patient's choice but continue to visit frequently. The team members will need to support each other.

Patient in denial

Unfortunately 'denial' has grown to have a rather negative connotation in health care. This attitude may potentially lead to harm. Denial is often used as a powerful protective mechanism, frequently allowing the patient to come to terms with a difficult situation in their own time. Shattering this denial is likely to expose a rawness that might not be able to bear exposure. Careful handling is therefore necessary.

The danger for the palliative care team member is the feeling that other health care professionals think that you should be able to help the patient (or the relative) face up to their problems. If you don't, you might even be seen to be colluding with the denial. However, attempts at trying to understand how much the patient or relative should know should be approached carefully. It is often better to find other ways of establishing a relationship of trust, for example meeting a need that is unrelated to the diagnosis. It is important not to push too hard but to wait for an opportune moment. Sometimes, the opportunity will be lost, for example the patient goes home, or the relative only visits in the evening. If this is the case, other health professionals need to be alerted and supported in the task of respecting the patient until such time that the truth can be acknowledged. For some patients, this never occurs.

Hydration and nutrition in the terminal phase

There cannot be a blanket policy on the issue of hydration and nutrition in the terminal phase of an illness. The decision must be based on an assessment of the risks and benefits. If a patient has been vomiting severely or there is a problem with hypercalcaemia then it would be a legitimate and appropriate decision to commence intravenous fluids. However, artifical hydration for dying patients does not prolong survival (NHCSPCS 1993;. Dunphy *et al.* 1995). Thirst is not usually a problem in patients dying of cancer, possibly because the cytokines produced from the tumour reduce the sensation of thirst (R. J. Dunlop, personal communication—paper awaiting publication). In these patients, intravenous fluids may even be harmful, causing peripheral and pulmonary oedema.

For relatives sitting with a patient who is dying over several days, issues about hydration (and occasionally nutrition) can sometimes cause anxiety. It is often helpful for you to raise the subject and help talk through some of the points with them. Often families are unaware of the complications of giving fluids in the last few days of life. They can be encouraged to give sips of fluid and moisten the mouth. If a decision is taken to give subcutaneous fluids then it should be reviewed on a day-to-day basis.

The issue of nasogastric feeding for patients with a major stroke who are unable to communicate their wishes can be difficult. If the patient is not elderly, the dying process can sometimes be quite prolonged. Such a situation might justify the use of nasogastric feeding. The ultimate decision needs to be made by the senior doctor on the team, but always taking into account what the family may be thinking and feeling towards their loved one. More often than not nature takes its course with a static pneumonia despite a nasogastric tube in place. The palliative care team can find out what the family's wishes are and can support them as they cope with the uncertainty of the illness.

Parenteral nutrition is more debatable. The literature shows that parenteral nutrition appears to have a role in well-selected patients. However, selection of patients varies widely from country to country because of patient and family expectations, costs, and culture (Fainsinger 1997). In general, parenteral nutrition is of value if the patient has treatable disease. There is no evidence that parenteral nutrition increases life expectancy in patients with advanced, untreatable disease. It may even accelerate cancer growth.

Euthanasia

There is no doubt that the whole issue of euthanasia is a highly personal one; yet, as part of the health-care team caring for patients and their families, we are considerably affected by such requests and there is growing pressure for us to have an opinion on the subject. A patient's decision for euthanasia affects not only themselves but also their families and the professionals involved in caring for them. Within the acute hospital such a request can be very unnerving for those who are not accustomed to the debate nor to such a request.

The debate surrounding euthanasia has widened since the setting up of the Euthanasia Society of Great Britain in the 1930s. In those days the debate was generally confined to patients facing an often painful and lingering form of death from advanced cancer (Saunders 1980). Nowadays it includes patients with severe non-malignant conditions such as multiple sclerosis, the young quadriplegic, the elderly invalid, the senile, and even those suffering from chronic psychiatric disease.

Wilkes *et al.* (1993), in their small study looking at nurses' attitudes towards euthanasia and its effect on relationships in the workplace in Australia and Hong Kong, found little difference between the cultures. Much of this appeared to be due to the lack of any debate, and even of education on the moral and ethical issues, surrounding the subject. Not being prepared for a request for euthanasia by a patient can cause considerable anxiety in an overstretched ward team. As specialists in palliative care, we need to be aware of the different arguments and issues involved.

In Holland, Professor Van der Maas and colleagues (1991) carried out a nationwide retrospective study to look at the incidence of active euthanasia. They give the following reasons why patients had requested euthanasia:

- loss of dignity   57%
- pain   46%
- unworthy dying   46%
- dependency on others   33%
- tiredness of life   23%.

Interestingly, Chochinov *et al.* (1995) prospectively investigated the prevalence of the desire for death in 200 terminally ill patients in the US. A desire for death to come sooner was common (44.5% of patients), with 8.5% patients acknowledging a longing to die. This latter group's desire for death correlated with ratings of pain and low family support but most significantly with measures of depression. However, when the depression was treated the desire of death abated. Chochinov *et al.* argue that treatable problems were present in a large majority of those desiring death. When symptoms and issues about care within a terminal illness are not resolved, it would appear that the desire to end life is heightened.

When faced with a request for euthanasia, the focus of the mind and emotions of the healthcare professional is sharpened. This demand from the patient can have different effects on the way health professionals react. Either they do not know how to handle such a request and so find it difficult to engage in conversation for fear of the subject being brought up again, or it has the completely opposite effect of drawing the health professional into an unusually close relationship with the patient.

Oxenham and Boyd (1997) have succinctly detailed seven points that help discuss the topic of euthanasia with a patient.

1. It is important to be prepared to ask patients about possible thoughts of euthanasia. They use the analogy of a psychiatrist asking a depressed patient whether they have thoughts of suicide—lots of depressed patients do not, but those who do often find it helpful to talk about their feelings.
2. For those patients who request euthanasia, such a statement must be acknowledged and not avoided. It can so often be a cry for understanding and help.
3. Investigating the reasons behind such a request helps one to tangibly open up such a conversation rather than shy away.
4. More often than not there is opportunity to correct errors of perception. It may be that a request stems from a fear of dying in

pain because of seeing a close relative or friend die in pain, or a lack of understanding of the disease process and the fear of months and months of dependence. Just because one reason has been uncovered does not automatically mean that that is the only reason. Often it is important to ask 'is there anything else?'

5. A patient requesting euthanasia must be reassured that he or she still has control of treatment decisions. Just because one is dying should not mean loss of control with decisions being made behind one's back. It is important for team members to advocate with the patient's doctors or consultant that necessary information is shared in order for the patient to feel in control.

6. It can be helpful to explore aspects of spiritual pain (Hockley 1993). Just because the palliative care team has been asked to be involved does not mean that the team member has to come up with answers.

7. Often admitting one's own powerlessness to bring about a solution but at the same time acknowledging the situation can be extremely helpful in itself.

The last chapter of a book strikes a vivid analogy to the last chapter of one's life. Such a chapter may often not be very exciting, but it is where the essence of what has gone before is brought to a meaningful close. So too with the last few weeks or months of a life. Within today's society there seems to be an increasing danger that once a person loses the physical and social dimension to their life, life becomes pointless, empty, and without purpose. There is a desire to close the book before the story is finished. The terminal phase of an illness can, however, sometimes be an opportunity for the psychological and spiritual aspects to become more focused. For many, experience in tapping the psychological and spiritual strengths of one's life is limited, and sometimes non-existent within a family situation. Help is needed to highlight the significance of what is happening. Opportunity needs to be given in order that fears can be expressed, or just to sit and talk about real issues—the fear of impending death, the importance of past memories, the uncertainty of the dying process, the opportunity to make amends if communication has broken down for some reason.

By going through these steps, most patients who request early death are relieved. The remaining patients are often quite unemotional and rational. They continue to request euthanasia (Hockley 1993). Their rationality usually cannot be disputed, as they remain adamant in their reasoned request. These patients do not like uncertainty—the dying process represents the greatest loss of control. The alternative is to demand euthanasia; their reason is that 'dying is not living'. Our response is to affirm the request but to remind the patient that a lethal injection is not possible. The patient can be offered repeat doses of a sedative if the suffering becomes unbearable. This usually restores the sense of control.

Summary

Ethical decisions often arise in the care of terminally ill patients. Complex problems involve the patient, the family, and the health care professionals. Palliative care teams are often called on to support the staff. Team members need to have a clear understanding of the ethical basis for making decisions. They need to have considered issues such as euthanasia. The support of other team members is vital in these situations. The next chapter deals with team dynamics.

6

Team dynamics

Palliative care teams are subject to a number of forces, from both within and outside the team. Team members frequently feel pulled in several directions. Only by working together as a team, supporting, encouraging, and learning from one another, will the necessary sense of competence and self-confidence be maintained in order to enjoy the work, grow as individuals, and provide a dynamic service.

In the last 20 years the number of hospital-based multidisciplinary palliative care teams in the UK has increased from two in 1977 to 139 listed in the 1997 St Christopher's Hospice Directory, London. However, the life span of some teams has been short (Herxheimer *et al.* 1985)—testimony to the potentially destructive strength of destabilizing forces. If a team is to survive, these forces must be recognized and reduced. Balancing forces are needed to maintain the integrity of the individuals and the team.

This chapter seeks to examine the dynamics of palliative care teams. Broadly speaking, the forces acting on a team are derived from influences outside the team (environmental factors), and from interactions within the team itself (internal factors). We have chosen to weave these factors into a sequence, commencing with 'how the team works' in relation to the hospital setting—establishing goals at the inception of the team, working with patients and families, what to do if advice is declined. The second part of the chapter discusses the interactions between team members, role blurring, the effect of the work on individuals within the team, leadership of a team, how to recognize and manage conflict within the team, and fulfiling the educational needs of team members.

Team goals

'Team' is more than a descriptive term for a collection of individuals with a common geographic base. Beckhard (1974) recognized that a team is a functional dynamic entity 'a group with a specific task or tasks, the accomplishment of which requires the interdependent and collaborating efforts of its members'.

The cohesion of a specialist palliative care team will require the members to agree upon, and be committed to, a common set of goals which address the needs of patients, families, and staff. The goals outlined in Chapter 1 were based on these needs, and therefore bear repeating:

- To work alongside the ward team caring for terminally patients by advising on symptom control and psychosocial/existential issues.
- To provide extra counselling and support to relatives finding difficulties with more complex grief situations.
- To provide support and advice to the staff caring for these patients.
- To take part in multidisciplinary education relating to issues of palliative care:
  - informally at ward level
  - formal lectures
  - writing of booklets or guidelines
- Act as liaison between the hospital and existing hospices/home care services
- To audit and research areas of interest such as symptom control or issues surrounding the emotional impact of dying.

These goals emphasize a broad approach encompassing psychosocial and medical needs. They maintain the focus on the importance of a multidisciplinary approach. Medical problems cannot then become the priority, as is characteristic of the biomedical model.

Goals need to be adapted to the specific situation, taking into account the other services that exist in the hospital or local district. The care of bereaved relatives may be best incorporated into local services such as Cruse (a national UK bereavement organization), although some teams run their own bereavement support service.

The hospital palliative care team is often developed after hospice in-patient and home care services. The setting up of a team in the acute setting can be unsettling, especially when the other services in the area have been established many years. It is sometimes difficult for established services to re-set their own goals to allow for a new specialist palliative care service within the hospital. For example, specialist home care nurses who have been used to coming into the hospital need to realize that their visits may not need to be so frequent; that time previously spent visiting the hospital can now be usefully re-directed toward teaching district nurses in a local health centre. Diplomacy is needed in working through the decisions. Establishing goals and boundaries can take time and a great deal of patience. If, however, there is no nearby home care service, the palliative care team may wish to extend their role outside the hospital. The teaching role will depend on the educational input of the local hospice, universities, and hospital in-service education.

Setting limits

It is rare that a specialist palliative care service within a hospital starts as a fully established multidisciplinary team. Setting limits is therefore very important. Needless to say this can be extremely frustrating, but it is important to hold to.

One of the key factors in establishing an effective team is perseverance of the original team member(s), if possible for the first 5 years of the service. If the team is to develop without casualties along the way, team members need to conserve their energy without losing the vision. Specific limits may be built into team objectives. Several teams restrict their services to only seeing terminally ill cancer patients. However, there is greater pressure to be involved with patients dying of non-malignant disease, in the hope of disseminating hospice philosophy to other specialties. Occasionally, teams limit patient or family involvement to a single review, with the primary team responsible for follow-up rather than providing continuous support throughout a terminal illness.

Patients with benign pain are often referred, particularly if there is no pain clinic. The palliative care team should have a consistent policy for these patients. On-going care may require a limit to the length of involvement, particularly when patients are undergoing curative treatment or have early disease. 'Pending' patients from the current list is appropriate as long as they are given a card or some means of contacting the team if necessary in the future.

Geographic boundaries need to be clearly defined. This is particularly important if other teams border on or work within the district. For small teams working solely in the hospital, it may be helpful to have boundaries within the hospital and only cover one or two directorates until more staff have been appointed. A limit may be established by concentrating on educational issues rather than carrying a full clinical load. There is no doubt that clinical work is very satisfying, but it is also extremely time consuming when a team is short of personnel.

It can be difficult to try to set limits once a team has become well known. However, this may be necessary, especially when the team is faced with a period of lack of personnel through resignation or sickness.

Measuring goals

Goals need to be attainable, and team members should be able to appreciate when they have achieved them. Otherwise, uncertainty and dissatisfaction will result. Many symptoms, particularly pain, can be controlled; the positive feedback from patients and families provides a measure of success as well as a powerful reward.

Formally measuring specialist palliative care intervention is important not only for the team's confidence but also as a proof to the hospital board that the team is competent. Many teams have become involved in evaluating projects to audit effectiveness, and identify areas of care that need to be improved. Scales for rating severity of symptoms during chemotherapy may be readily adapted. Several workers (Kristjanson 1986; MacAdam and Smith 1987) are developing easily administered questionnaires which also assess emotional, social, and spiritual needs of patients and families. Symptom check-lists completed by patients (McCorkle and Young *et al.* 1978; Bruera *et al.* 1991) at the bedside can be a useful way of auditing the effect of actual practice. The STAS tool (Higginson *et al.* 1992) has been used both by solo nurse specialists and by palliative care teams to measure their effectiveness. Ellershaw *et al.* (1995) developed the PACA instrument measuring three aspects of intervention by a specialist palliative care team:

- patient's symptom control
- patient's and family's understanding of progression of disease
- placement.

It is important to keep records and compile statistics about workloads. Demonstrating an increase in the number of referrals, visits, home deaths, teaching commitments, and transfers to hospice may help to consolidate the team's position. This information will be needed for any business case to expand the team.

Another measure of effectiveness is the decreased number of complaints about the care of the dying. This is readily appreciated by the hospital administration (Hockley *et al.* 1988). Postive feedback from other staff is very important, but will not readily be forthcoming initially. In time, it becomes another significant source of job satisfaction.

Patient referrals to the team

From the outset, it is important to define the way in which referrals are made to the team. Nurses frequently want to refer patients; they are more likely to be aware of the problems. However, the consultant must give permission for specialist palliative care involvement. It is the consultant who has overall clinical responsibility for the patient. It is therefore only polite that the ward nurse discusses involving the palliative care team with the consultant or senior doctor in charge. When referrals are initiated by the ward nurses alone, a palliative care team can become inundated with new patients so that often more indepth conversations are not tackled because of the workload. This situation arises particularly where a nurse specialist is working alone. It is important to keep in mind that the palliative care team in the acute hospital is not there to see all terminally ill patients but just those with particular problems or difficulties.

Confirmation of consent therefore must be given before the patient is seen, particularly if the primary team has never used the palliative care team before. Failure to observe this principle will lead to embarrassment and stress, even jeopardize the future use of the team. Confirmation can be established in a number of ways:

- by using a referral form
- by the referring doctor requesting specialist advice by writing in the medical notes
- by contacting a member of the palliative care team by telephone.

A referral form can be a useful audit tool, especially if the reason for referral is documented. A team member can then compare the reason for referral with the problems that the patient and family identify. If these forms are made up on a pad they are less likely to get lost or put away in a filing cabinet where no one can find them. When first establishing a service, referring medical staff should write in the medical notes to request specialist advice, even if this changes once the team is established. Eventually the most common way of referring a patient to an established palliative care team is by telephoning the request through to the office or team member.

Initial details of how to make a referral to the palliative care team can be printed on a sheet of A4paper and sent to each ward, nurse manager, consultant, and clinical director that the service wants to cover.

The profile that the palliative care team maintains on the wards will influence the number and stage of referrals. Informal visits to wards will frequently prompt staff to seek advice or refer a patient sooner. This reduces the stress of late referrals but increases the workload. Conversely, involvement with home care will limit the time available to spend on the wards and might jeopardize establishing the team within the hospital. Also if a team is predominantly involved in community visits, patients may only be referred when they are about to be discharged.

How palliative care teams relate to patients and families

Initial visits

The palliative care team will need to plan how patient referrals will be reviewed. The initial interview is best conducted by someone with experience in symptom control; approximately two thirds of the authors' patients are referred because of distressing symptoms. It is not unusual to find that many patients referred for psychosocial support also have unrecognized distressing symptoms. The nurse specialists usually see most of the patients, particularly when the doctor works part-time. The doctor will then follow up the initial visit if necessary.

The person with the lowest case load, or least complicated cases, will often see the new referral; some negotiation between team members may be required. Occasionally, circumstances will favour a specific member reviewing a new patient. Being invited to see a new patient can cause some anxiety. This may be more of a problem for the nurse specialist (especially if he or she is the first member to be appointed on the team or is new to the team) than for the team doctor.

- How to introduce oneself?
- Is there anything more that can be offered that hasn't already been suggested?

These are some of the difficulties. Generally, patients will have been told by the ward team that they are to be referred to the palliative care team for advice. However, it is good to check. Introducing yourself is important, as the first visit can make all the difference. Some aspects of the team's role may be emphasized more than others, depending on what the patient understands about the disease. If pain or other symptoms cannot be used by way of introduction then a nurse specialist may well want to say something like

. . . I am a nurse specialist who works in the oncology unit. Your doctors have specifically asked me to come and see you regarding . . . support at home, the way you are feeling just now.

The initial visit is an important time and should not be hurried. Often patients take the opportunity in meeting somebody new to explore more deeply what they understand about their illness. If the visit is limited by time, interruptions, or a focusing on just physical symptoms then this opportunity is often lost, sometimes forever. If there is only a short time in which to see a new patient then a further appointment should be made for when more time is available.

A course of action may need to be confirmed immediately with the patient, particularly when symptoms are causing distress. Previous experience in palliative care will usually enable advice to be provided at the time. One should feel comfortable about asking another team member to come to the ward if there is uncertainty about the situation. The team should have a forum for discussing strategies for needs that are not so immediate (see page 101: 'Relating together as a team'). The experience of the Charing Cross Hospital Support Team illustrates the importance of the team members meeting together to make decisions. Failure in communication was one of the factors cited in the collapse of the team (Herxheimer *et al.* 1985).

It may be more appropriate for the doctor on the team to see patients with non-malignant conditions. A palliative care team member who has a good relationship with a difficult primary team should be considered for new referrals from that team. Some primary teams feel less threatened by nurses, others are more comfortable with a doctor. The person who conducts the initial interview often becomes the key worker for that patient. This provides a continuity that contrasts with the frequent changes in other staff. The nurses and doctors of the primary team find it helpful to know which member of the palliative care team to contact in the event of new problems. Occasional contacts with other members of the palliative care team minimize disruption of care when the key worker is sick or on holiday. If the social worker becomes the key worker, a nurse will often maintain a minimal contact; regular joint visits by the nurse and social worker may be appropriate with some patients.

Continuity of care is particularly important when a patient is transferred to another ward or primary team. The key worker can focus the attention of the new staff by telling them what has already happened to the patient and family. If more than one primary team is involved, it can be useful to identify for the patient and family which consultant is dealing with which problem.

Some palliative care teams prefer new patients to be seen by two team members. This has the advantage of providing different insights and perspectives about the patient's problems. There are also fewer difficulties when team members are absent for any reason. If only one team member is to carry out the initial interview then this opens up opportunity for a member of the ward team to be present if they have the time. In this way the ward nurse or doctor not only observes the interaction and hopefully learns from the experience, but also becomes more involved and likely to help implement what is suggested.

It is very important to establish limits on the number of referrals that are accepted. This will minimize role overload. Although it is difficult to generalize, an average of 3–4 new hospital referrals a week per full-time equivalent nurse or doctor on the team is probably a comfortable maximum. The nature of the case load will influence this; 3–4 difficult symptom control or psychosocial problems may be more taxing than 10 'straightforward' patients. Lunt and Hillier (1981) considered 60 new patients a year per nurse to be an ideal for home care. Our more recent experience has shown that after 4 years of gradually introducing a team (often only 3–4 specialists by this point) referrals often reach around 400 new patients a year within a 600-bedded teaching/university hospital.

Follow-up visits

The frequency of follow-up visits should be carefully considered. Patients can be seen every day but this may prove counterproductive. Ward doctors and nurses may reduce contact with the patient because they see the palliative care team involved so frequently. Most teams review in-patients 2–3 times a week on average. Patients with very distressing symptoms will be an exception; they may require review several times a day until their symptoms are brought under control.

The number of visits should enable sufficient time for the interviews to be relaxed and unhurried. It may take several visits before the patient opens up about their deepest fears and anxieties; they are accustomed to accepting symptoms and worries rather than interrupting the nurses' busy schedule or the doctors' hurried routine visits. You must show there is the time and the strength to accept their fears, anger, and grief.

Commitment to the patient is demonstrated by being reliable, visiting as promised and following up any requests from the patient. Facilitating consultations by visiting the surgeon or physician, or finding results of tests by visiting the laboratory or X-ray department, may also help.

Given that many patients die within weeks of referral, it is important to recognize the value of even one family session. Asking to see a family together is a statement of the team's concern and the family's importance. A family meeting can generate confidence in a situation that feels out of control. The session can be used to encourage family strengths, help them to identify and include other supports around them such as church, and address what is reasonable for them to expect of each other.

Out-patient contact

The out-patient contact can be a very satisfactory continuum of care both for the specialist team member and the patient. When patients attend clinics, the team member tries to see the patient before they go in to see the consultant or senior registrar. This helps to minimize the effect of delays. Accompanying the patient facilitates the interview and improves the quality of the contact with the doctors. If transport to the clinic is difficult, a volunteer scheme or a taxi service should be arranged rather than having the patient wait for hospital transport.

A more unpredictable aspect of out-patient work occurs when a team member is called to see a new patient in a clinic. This most commonly occurs when a palliative care team is well known within the hospital, especially in a cancer centre. It is difficult to resist such a request, despite the inconvenience; it is rare that a team member is called at a time when they are not involved in something that has to be cut short, or left, in order to meet this need. This situation often occurs when there are no beds available for admission. More often than not the patient and family are really pleased that someone has been able to come, but the interview can feel rushed and unsatisfactory. This situation is acceptable on an occasional basis but the referring doctor may need to be made aware that is not to be considered normal practice.

A few teams provide an out-patient clinic. These clinics are kept small, with only 6–7 patients attending one afternoon a week. This allows time for the patients and relatives to talk about their problems. It can be a better way for new patients to be seen in an out-patient clinic if they are well enough to wait for an appointment. Such clinics are usually only appropriate if there is a full-time doctor on the team.

When the number of referrals is overwhelming the resources on the team, then it may be that following up patients and their families in the different out-patient clinics has to be limited to those patients specifically requiring on-going support.

Patients value regular telephone contacts, especially if there is no specialist palliative care service in the community. If this is not maintained, patients may be re-admitted without the team knowing for several days. One solution could be the use of a sticker on the hospital notes which requests that the primary team contact the palliative care team immediately the patient is re-admitted.

Bereavement follow-up

Following the death of a patient, the relatives can be seen when they collect the death certificate and the patient's belongings. Different hospitals have different policies when it comes to collecting belongings. Some will give the clothes of the deceased and the death certificate to the relatives shortly after the death, especially if the family live a long way from the hospital. Others will ask relatives to come back the next day when a bereavement officer will deal with procedures. Whatever the hospital policy, it is important that a bereavement booklet explaining details of registering the death, the emotional impact of grief, helping children in their grief, suggested literature, and how to seek further help if necessary, is given to every deceased next-of-kin. Further contact can be maintained with the family by telephone call, letter, or follow-up visit.

Bereavement follow-up can be difficult because of the time required and the aesthetics of the hospital environment. One-to-one follow-up is perhaps the least labour intensive, with sessions being reserved for those highlighted as being 'at risk'. Often relatives want to talk to people who knew their loved one. This makes it difficult to refer to outside agencies or hospice bereavement services, especially when such agencies already have a waiting list. One-to-one sessions can therefore be a useful stop-gap. Any bereavement programme which is more sophisticated than this requires someone from the team to co-ordinate it.

Teams operating a more comprehensive follow-up programme usually have a social worker; few teams are fortunate enough to have the services of a bereavement coordinator and volunteers. Regular meetings for the bereaved can open discussion about coping with loss, adjusting to isolation, dealing with the disposal of clothing, going on holiday alone, family support, and gradually becoming independent.

Groups can be organized on a continuous monthly basis, or limited to a specific number of weekly sessions. In our experience a meeting once a week for a 6 week period works well. The intensity of this type of group counselling combined with the day-to-day stresses experienced by the team can be very taxing. Two members of the team need to be responsible for each group—generally the social worker will coordinate the sessions with team members taking it in turns to help run a group. Casualty and intensive care services may want to refer bereaved families.

The stress of working with patients and families

Working with terminally ill patients and families can be very stressful. Extremes of emotional reaction, especially anger and aggression, are very difficult to cope with. These emotions are predictable responses to the devastating impact of a terminal illness, but that does not make these reactions any easier to deal with, particularly when they are directed at the members of the team rather than the cancer.

Patients come from a variety of cultural, religious, and social backgrounds. This can make interpretation of their reactions more difficult, particularly if language barriers exist. Translators do not necessarily help, because they often share the same powerful cultural forces which inhibit dealing with distressing information. In addition, truth-telling may not be the norm in some cultures and considerable distress will occur if this is not respected.

Patients referred at the end of their illness are a source of considerable stress. Distressing symptoms make the patient seem alert but their relief will restore the patient to a state of dying peacefully. However, the distress of the relatives will increase because they perceive the change in the patient to be an attempt to accelerate death. The difficulty in dealing with these reactions is compounded by the brief time available, and the frustration of thinking the task would have been easier if the patient had been referred earlier.

Even for a team member who has practised palliative care for many years, there are still times when a patient or family situation will appear overwhelmingly difficult and scary even before the first visit. Often the question of what else can be offered can be almost paralysing; yet the being there, the walking alongside, can be just as effective in the right situation as masterly words or fancy symptom control measures.

Empowering hope (Herth 1990) and not giving false hope is extremely important in any palliative care situation. In the acute hospital setting the degree of compromise that one automatically adapts to can sharpen the importance of gentle truth-telling. Situations in which families, but not patients, are told the diagnosis are becoming less frequent as the trend towards truth-telling increases. However, it is very stressful when families and the primary team pursue a strategy of collusion, particularly if the patient is distressed by their ignorance and is asking for more information. Breaking collusion will provoke an intense reaction from the relatives. Patience, diplomacy, support, and interaction with patient and family are required to resolve these problems.

Occasionally good symptom control measures help patients appear to be better and live a little longer than initially anticipated. Families can become angry with the palliative care team for helping them to accept the impending loss of a loved one, only to have the patient recover for a time. A similar situation may occur when patients and families attempt to patch up chronic problems. Long-standing disagreements may be set aside in an effort to make the patient's final days as enjoyable as possible. If the illness becomes protracted, old tensions may be refuelled by the frustration of the patient not dying, and then directed at the team.

It is not always possible to control pain, breathlessness, and other distressing symptoms, particularly when medications cause unacceptable side-effects. Some patients and families will be angry at this failure, using the opportunity to displace anger about the illness. A sense of impotence and failure may be further heightened if it is felt that your 'expert' status has been weakened in the minds of the other staff.

Patient denial can also cause a sense of failure, especially if there is a strong feeling that a patient should accept their illness. Nonetheless, there can be major difficulties if the team perseveres in trying to undermine it. Quite apart from the extra suffering experienced by the patient, they can become angry and reject the team. This may inhibit doctors from referring other patients. Patients who exercise denial may go so far as to discontinue all medications, including painkillers, in the belief that they are cured. It is even more common to find patients who want any attempt at curative treatment. Anything less is totally unacceptable. Their desperation may lead them to press for radical treatments such as aggressive chemotherapy, even if there has been no previous response, or disfiguring surgery.

More recently, a great deal of importance has been given to patients dying at home. It is the authors' belief that to enable this to happen greater communication needs to be given to patients and families regarding end-of-life issues (see chapter 5). If patients and their families are to be able to cope with a death at home, then considerable work has to be engineered within the acute hospital setting enabled by the palliative care team. Who does this, how it is done and the risk of it backfiring are never easy to work through, but become clearer as team members learn to calmly support each other, the primary team and the patients and families.

Communicating advice to the primary team

We have now come to the point where, having discussed the issues with the patient, you must advise the primary team. If a ward team have already waited 24 hours since the referral, then they will generally be looking for immediate advice after seeing the patient. This can be a pressure which should be resisted if you are not sure about the advice to be given. It is important to confirm your thoughts on what is the best advice with another member of the palliative care team or a local specialist in palliative care if a team member is not available. Even taking half an hour off the ward to check the literature may be appropriate in some situations.

Written information in either the medical notes or medical notes *and* nursing care plans is the best way in communicating information. To write in medical notes can be intimidating for some nurse specialists, but it is important to persevere. The advice written should be clear and follow a logical pattern. An explanation on how much the patient understands about the cancer or how far the disease has progressed is important; this is followed by firstly detailing problems as seen by the patient including symptom problems, lack of insight, home and family difficulties; and secondly, the suggestions or plan of action. Passing advice on verbally can help to build a rapport and is especially necessary if prompt action is required. As the palliative care team becomes accepted, advice about minor alterations in medications or treatment will require only informal discussion with medical or nursing staff. Comments do not necessarily need to be written in the notes at each consultation. In some situations it may seem easier to pass on advice and run, allowing the referring team to make a decision whether to comply or not. However, a commitment to patient choice will usually compel team members to persist as the patient's advocate when advice is ignored. These occasions highlight the harsh reality of the advisory role.

Whether one writes in the nursing care plans will depend on time available, and the calibre of the nurses involved at ward level. Some ward nurses are more conscientious than others about documenting the verbal advice given in the nursing care plans. If there is any doubt (often highlighted just by working with the different wards) then written communication in both medical notes and nursing care plans will be important.

Both doctors and nurses often have difficulty asking for and accepting advice. This is partly due to a lack of training in teamwork. It also represents a conservative tendency designed to protect the patient from harmful treatments. The palliative care team will be treated like a new drug: something with therapeutic potential, yet to be realized, and side-effects which must be balanced against that potential. Unfortunately, primary teams often presume that the side-effects will include increased patient anxiety and fear, even before team members begin to function. These presumptions are inherent in the way some palliative care teams have initially been labelled 'death squad' or 'angel of death'.

Advice which is radically different from the thinking of the primary team should be discussed with the consultant or registrar. The more formal setting of a ward round can be used, but this may be very daunting. Many consultants or senior registrars can be approached before a ward round; they may be more receptive to new suggestions which might otherwise be rejected in the more public setting of the round.

It is very tempting for the palliative care team doctor to expedite treatment changes by writing prescriptions. However, this will rob the referring doctors of a valuable teaching experience. It may take more time and effort to contact the junior doctor but greater dividends will result. Rarely, the doctor on the palliative care team may need to prescribe because the other staff are occupied in the operating theatre or 'on-call'.

When a referring team is approached for the first time, the referring doctors may well rigorously question advice given, particularly in teaching hospitals. If you have trained in hospice, where there is mutual agreement about treatments, it will be very disconcerting when evidence to support the advice is demanded, esoteric side-effects are pointed out, or alternatives are put forward. The interrogation is not designed to attack the team member but to serve as a reminder of who is responsible for the patient. In this situation, one must resist manufacturing answers for the sake of preserving credibility; a simple 'I do not know' will have more impact. Knowing that the advice represents a team consensus will give you more confidence, as will the company of another team member.

It is always important to remember that ward doctors and nurses are often under considerable pressure. If the reaction to advice is brisk, it is easy to fall into the trap of feeling paranoid that the response relates to the advice given. There may be factors that are feeding into a difficult day other than the palliative care team's advice! With time, most doctors will relax as they become aware of the efficacy and non-judgemental nature of the palliative care team. However, further challenges should be expected whenever the registrars or housestaff change-over. Palliative care teams are a reasonably new concept and not all doctors have had opportunity to work in hospitals where such a service exists. Being friendly and outgoing to new staff, even though a team member may feel under pressure with work, will help facilitate communication at a later date.

Attending ward rounds or multidisciplinary meetings, even when not involved with patients, can be a very valuable way to break down suspicions that the team feel they are somehow better than everyone else. It is also a good way to extend your own knowledge base in a specialist area not previously known by a team member. However, not every ward round can be attended and it is often only possible to go to one such meeting a week. Informal meetings over lunch can also have a similar effect. After a while, questions about terminal care will be asked, and patients may be referred.

Some problems lie outside the collective experience of the team, such as a difficult anxiety state that may need psychiatric consultation or a specific symptom problem that requires a more expert opinion. You should recognize these limitations and not be afraid to seek the advice of others. It can be particularly helpful to discuss problems with the local hospice, or a major teaching hospice. Pride may make this process difficult within the hospital. However, any fear of appearing incompetent must be set aside. Other staff may provide useful suggestions, and they appreciate the chance to be involved in this way. They will actually feel more comfortable about using the team. Even if the advice is not totally appropriate, the communication between both parties can only help raise the profile of the terminally ill. It is important to remember those professionals who are prepared to consider the plight of the terminally ill and who may therefore be of help in the future.Even though a problem remains unsolved and all possibilities exhausted, patients, family, and staff will still benefit from ongoing support. However, a key worker is likely to become worn down by frustration and disappointment, especially if the illness is protracted. Other team members should share the load by becoming involved with the patient and family.

What to do if advice is declined

If the advice of the palliative care team member is declined or ignored, the suffering of the patient and family may continue unabated. This can be extremely upsetting, particularly when the unnecessary suffering is contrasted with the dignity of patients in hospice. It is even more disturbing when a patient's anguish is increased by the team protesting about the failure to act on recommendations. Challenging the primary team may generate anger which is displaced onto the patient, either directly or by avoiding the patient.

The realization that the team may be responsible, even in a small part, for an increase in suffering can be very depressing and demoralizing. These emotions may exceed the usual feelings of anger and frustration. The team member will be left with a sense of only having a token role, with nothing to balance the loss of familiar skills, such as performing 'hands on' care, upon joining the palliative care team. When confronted by this situation, a decision must be made whether to persevere or not. It may be better to opt out from the care of that patient situation altogether, particularly if feelings are so intense that they are likely to spill over when talking to the primary team. Support from colleagues will be necessary whether you stay involved or not.

If you remain involved, it is important to try to determine why the primary team have not accepted the advice. Doctors usually make decisions based on what they feel is 'best for the patient'. This paternalistic approach is supported by case law. The right of the patient to make an informed judgement about his treatment has only received minority support from the legal profession (Sidaway v. Bethlem Board of Governors 1985). Currently, 'a doctor is not guilty of negligence if he has acted in accordance with a practice accepted as proper by a reasonable body of medical men skilled in that particular art' (Bolam v. Friern Hospital Management Committee). This principle, the Bolam principle, encompasses 'the practice of saying very little and waiting for questions from the patient' (Bolam v. Friern Hospital Management Committee).

These medico-legal considerations mean that some doctors must be assured that advice is based on 'accepted' practice before they will accept it. It is possible to reverse some decisions if evidence from the literature can be provided. This underlines the importance of knowing about key papers on different aspects of palliative care.

The paternalistic basis for decisions frequently reflects a genuine altruistic response. You can appeal to such charitable motives by presenting more personal details which help the doctors realize they are dealing with a person rather than a 'case'. Less commonly, paternalism signifies a rigid authoritarian position. This attitude is the most difficult to influence. In this situation, alternative strategies should be developed which can facilitate a compromise:

- consider asking another member of the palliative care team to take over the case
- does the consultant or senior registrar involved find it easier to relate to a doctor or a team member of a different sex?
- try to realize that if you were not involved then the patient would not be having any different care anyway
- would the consultant listen more easily to the ward sister?

If advice is initially rejected, wait and see if anything changes. It is surprising how often the primary team will subsequently alter the patient's treatment. The change is often a compromise in favour of the suggestions rather than whole-hearted acceptance. For example, the primary team might increase subtherapeutic parenteral doses of pethidine (meperidine) rather than change to oral morphine. Any efforts in the right direction should be praised. The best way to do this is to tell the primary team that the patient is grateful for the improvement in pain control. You can then mention that the patient is still in pain and ask if they would consider increasing the dose and frequency.

Negotiating around what is familiar to the primary team will usually produce a more satisfactory result for the patient, but the reader will appreciate that the compromise may involve the patient continuing to experience distressing symptoms. Such a compromise is never ideal. The stress may be lessened by recognizing some progress will have been made, if not for the patient in question, then for subsequent patients. It is the degree of compromise which you can accept that will determine whether you can continue to work in this advisory role.

When advice is declined the alternative of not talking directly to the primary team may seem very attractive. You might try to use the nursing or junior medical staff to pass on your comments. Unfortunately this only increases the stress of the ward staff as they find themselves caught in the middle of the palliative care team and consultant or senior registrar. Progress is even less likely when this happens.

Finally, if you feel that you are getting nowhere with a situation it might be possible to suggest transferring the patient to a hospice. Clearly this depends on how willing the patient is about the idea.

It is extremely difficult to keep visiting a patient when advice has been declined and the patient is still suffering. The team member can feel particularly impotent not only towards the primary team but also in front of the patient. Unfortunately, these difficulties are not easy to hide and there is a considerable danger of the patient feeling obliged to keep the peace.

Other stresses on a palliative care team

Hospital services

The expectations that primary teams have about the palliative care team may produce considerable strain. Many consultants hold the view that the function of a palliative care team is to transfer patients to a hospice. This view arises from the clinician's dilemma when there are delays in potentially curable cancer operations because of a shortage of acute beds. The pressure can seriously undermine the ability of the palliative care team to establish a rapport with the patient. Many patients will welcome the opportunity to go to a hospice; it is important to recognize these patients quickly so that they can benefit from early transfer. Others will be extremely upset. The consultant may respond to a special plea, especially if the nursing staff on the ward support the patient's choice. On the few occasions when a reversal of the decision has not been obtained, the patients have died very quickly after transfer (Dunlop and Hockley 1991)

Similarly, there is often great pressures for the team to get involved the day before a patient is due to be discharged. These patients are often still symptomatic but the referring team are adamant the patient should be discharged. Another slightly different example is the urgent Friday afternoon referral. It may be that in both these situations the referral should be refused. Nonetheless both scenarios can be a risk both to the patient and to future referrals from that particular team.

Problems also arise when terminally ill patients or relatives request readmission to hospital. If the patient is well known to a ward, this can often be arranged easily. However, lack of acute beds on the ward may require the patient to be admitted via Accident and Emergency or a 'holding' ward. The admitting team or emergency staff may be angry and obstruct the admission, even discharge the patient. Terminally ill patients are not yet considered emergencies, even though their weakened state magnifies the intensity of symptoms and the distress of relatives. Where possible, the nurse specialist should arrange to meet the patient and family in the Accident and Emergency Department and accompany them to the ward.

Community services

Hospital palliative care teams working with general practitioners and district nurses will find that the advisory role can be just as difficult in the community. Many problems, such as reluctance to use strong opioid painkillers, are similar to the hospital setting. These problems are compounded by the suspicions about hospital-based staff encroaching into the community. Diplomacy and flexibility are just as necessary for overcoming these fears.

Occasionally it is necessary to visit in the community despite a particular palliative care team's remit being confined to the hospital. If such a visit is necessary then it is probably best to inform the family physician and/or community nurse if for any reason they are not already aware of the difficulty. Sometimes a case conference in the health centre can help to clarify the difficulties without it being necessary to visit the home. Inviting one of the community team to accompany you on the home visit can also ease any concerns.

Hospices, hospice home care teams and other local hospital palliative care specialists

Hospital palliative care teams will frequently need to liaise with local hospices, their respective home care teams, and/or local specialist nurses. In general, liaison should not be difficult particularly if you have allayed misapprehensions during the planning of the team.

The team should be aware of the specific limitations in other services. Smaller hospice units will have difficulty taking in patients for more than 2–3 weeks respite care. Some hospices and home care services will only take patients in the final weeks of life. Problems may arise with 'shared care'; working with patients who are still receiving active treatment may be unacceptable to some hospices.

It is always helpful to make time to meet together. This can break down barriers and suspicions about each other's role. It will also foster a sense of working together as specialists in palliative care within that district. Different types of meetings can be arranged, for example to discuss ideas on research and audit. Other meetings might be more patient orientated or supportive in nature.

Lectures and visitors

Education is clearly high on the agenda of most specialists working in palliative care teams (see chapter 3). Many people find the exhilaration and feedback of teaching provides an important source of job satisfaction and motivation to the work. Although preparation of lectures takes time and has to be done out of working hours, the process of preparing and giving the lecture is stimulating. For those who enjoy this, it has a reviving effect which counters the draining of emotional energy often experienced with patient and family work.

However, limits need to be established or the service to patients may suffer. If a team member is always away giving lectures and not available to carry their portion of referrals, then tension will be created within the team.

The same inter-role conflict can occur if too many visitors are allowed to visit the team. Nowadays, postgraduate courses often lead to frequent requests to spend time with a team. These requests should be channelled through the main business meeting or at least discussed with the appropriate team members before being confirmed. More than one or two visitors per week can be very disruptive to the cohesion of the team and also to the welfare of patients being visited by the team.

Relating together as a team

The first part of this chapter has considered how palliative care teams relate to some of the external forces on the team. This next part now addresses the internal aspects of team building. The importance of relating together as a team across different professional backgrounds cannot be over-emphasized. This requires an understanding of the dynamics of small groups. Obviously communication is a major issue. It is how we communicate with each other at various meetings and how we relate to each other in the everyday clinical work that will reflect the cohesiveness and strength of the team. So often a team can become almost like a family, where we expect to understand intuitively, to be accepted, and to feel at home. We often forget that to grow together as a group involves discipline, openness, and sensitivity. After examining clinical meetings, business meetings, and team reviews (an opportunity to vocalize stressors and discuss future aspects of team life), there is a section on leadership followed by a reflection on one palliative care team's experience.

Clinical meetings

Regular clinical meetings provide the clinical supervision and support necessary to make decisions on complex cases. Since many of the referrals to a palliative care team are complex and require specialist opinion, there has to be some regular, multidisciplinary forum for discussion to take place. Ideally this meeting should happen once a day. The best time of day is for the team to decide; it will depend on both the size and composition of the team and the environment in which it works.

Clinical meetings should become a forum for presenting any new patients seen the day before, as well as ongoing complex problems encountered with patients or families. Discussing a difficult situation with other team members in a formal meeting will often make the problems become clearer and identify a way forward. This form of clinical supervision is especially helpful for the nurse specialists. The meetings should, however, be kept strictly to time.

The traditional medical model requires the doctor to be the leader of such meetings. This has important consequences for the dynamics. 'Leader' is usually synonymous with 'decision-maker'. Decisions will tend to be made on a unilateral basis, or by default if non-medical staff feel compelled to stay quiet when they disagree. Occasionally, this will lead to team members lacking the commitment necessary to action decisions. The nurse specialists will be less confident about making urgent decisions at the patient's bedside if the doctor makes all the decisions at these meetings. Difficulties will also arise if the doctor is frequently unavailable, or new members of the team want a greater role in the decision-making process.

Some teams may wish to develop beyond the traditional model. It takes a lot of effort to break down conventional, status-determined patterns. The observations and opinions of all team members must be affirmed and valued; too often, praise is considered inappropriate for professionals doing a job. Senior team members, particularly the doctor, should be sure that they do not cut short information from other team members. The aim should be to build up a variety of strategies based on collective experience, rather than the 'right' way. This model has more flexibility for dealing with complex non-medical problems.

Most teams have at least one regular meeting a week to discuss new patients and ongoing problems. These meetings concentrate the variety of disciplines and individual talents of the members. Problem definition is greatly enhanced and several perspectives can be generated. Such meetings take on a wider perspective and peripheral members of the team can be invited, i.e. chaplain, psychiatrist, oncologist, occupational therapist, physiotherapist, pharmacist. Obviously the dynamics of this meeting with both core and peripheral team members is different. The meeting is longer and more formal, often lasting a couple of hours. Useful information can be gained from the psychiatrist, oncologist, or anaesthetist who are committed to attending this weekly meeting. Occasionally it may be appropriate to invite other health professionals involved in a particularly complex patient/family scenario to this meeting if a decision has not been resolved at a ward round.

Team meetings

Team or business meetings help to organize a team that responds to individual needs, priorities and responsibilities. With different professionals being involved in the team, individuals will be asked to take part in educational days, seminars, etc. It is important that the team responds to such requests together and that there is a forum where such things can be discussed and different duties delegated.

A business meeting should probably occur every other week. Every effort must be made to make sure that no other meeting, teaching engagements, etc. clash. It is important that issues and topics for discussion are raised either prior to the meeting or as the meeting starts. The meeting can begin with examining the team diary and co-ordinating the various commitments of team members. Issues such as visitors to the team, conferences being attended, the need to respond to a recent journal article, and ways to make the team more effective can be raised and thought through together.

Team reviews

Team reviews serve as a forum for stress and conflict management. They should be a regular feature of team life, remaining distinct from the daily and weekly or biweekly team meetings described above. It is up to the team how often a review meeting should take place. The important factor is regularity. Obviously any review meeting being set up should be discussed with current team members. Some teams meet every 2 weeks and may include discussion about aspects of team function before opening up into the more nitty gritty aspects of team life; this may a less threatening way of starting review meetings. Other teams will make it solely a review time and meet monthly, even taking either a half day or whole day out of their work routine.

These review meetings can be facilitated in a variety of ways, depending on how team members want to use them. A few teams make use of an 'objective' facilitator, i.e. a psychologist or social worker who is experienced at facilitating small group work. This person is not normally part of the team. One team uses a management group comprising a community physician, director of nursing services, senior hospital social worker, and chaplain to handle problems and personal matters. The group meets regularly with the palliative care team. Other teams facilitate their own time. No one way is better and the group together need to develop what is right for them. Such a meeting is designed to help not hinder the group. It may be that a 'review meeting' is one of the last meetings to become regularly established, especially if the palliative care team is evolving over a number of years.

For review meetings to be useful, team members should become familiar with the causes and manifestations of stress within themselves and their colleagues. Vachon's reviews (1986, 1987) of stress and the care of the dying are highly recommended. Some stress may be valuable as a stimulus to better performance. However, when coping mechanisms are over-whelmed, physical symptoms, such as fatigue, weight change, and sleep disturbance may develop. Feelings of guilt, anger, irritability, and frustration will generate conflicts in the team and the individual's private life. If stress continues unabated, confidence will be undermined, and the team member will experience difficulty in making or implementing decisions. Eventually, depression and a sense of helplessness will render the individual incapable of continuing in their job.

The initial reviews will often consist of sharing anxieties about being exposed in the advisory role. The stresses inherent in coming to terms with new roles, a new environment, and a new set of colleagues will be submerged by the excitement of embarking on a new venture, and the need to build up a sense of 'being in it together'. Eventually, the 'honeymoon' excitement that sustains team members during the initial months will wane. The reality of trying to meet the needs of the dying and their carers will become starkly apparent, as will any mismatch between team members' skills and job requirements. The impact of patient deaths will hit home, particularly for team members who have not worked in hospice. Review sessions will be characterized by the venting of frustrations about people outside the team—the 'uncooperative' doctors, 'unfeeling' nurses, and 'ungrateful' patients.

As time progresses, team members will become increasingly aware of personality and professional conflicts within the team. The usual tendency is to suppress disagreement and conflict because there is a need to have the team's approval and the reaffirmation that you are nice and doing the right thing. It is important to recognize that 'chronic niceness' (each team member wearing a smiling mask that hides ill-feeling) may be very important for the functional integrity of the team, at least in the short term. However, there are problems with maintaining a facade. Team members may also sublimate personal conflict into their job. Expending mental energy to maintain an illusion of team cohesion will detract from performing clinical tasks and, in the end, the fragility of team relationships will buckle under the emotional strain. Tension may be eased by discussing the situation with others on the team but not with the person who is perceived to be the cause of the conflict. This may work in the short term, but has the long-term effect of creating factions and further disruption. Releasing tensions after work will disrupt relationships with family and friends.

Taking down the masks of 'chronic niceness' is very difficult. It can take several months before safety within the team permits the exploring of disagreements. Criticism will be perceived as a personal attack and will result in loss of self-esteem. It is vital to build up an atmosphere of trust and mutual respect by recognizing and encouraging team member's skills and strengths. This can be done by sharing personal successes and achievements at a team level, and allowing others to give due praise. For some this may not be easy, especially if their personality does not acknowledge their successes. This affirmation has to be realistic and not paternalistic. In a supportive atmosphere, constructive solutions can be explored if job mismatch is exposed. It may be appropriate to alter the job description to suit the team member better or encourage the learning of new skills. In some cases, situations which exacerbate the problem should be avoided; occasionally this may necessitate leaving the job.

Obviously it is the aim of every team not only to be effective but to relate well with those on the team itself. It would seem that the two have to be synonymous. However, because team members have different personalities, come from different backgrounds, and have different roles it is not always as easy as one would wish. Characteristics of effective teams appear to incorporate both the relating within the team and communicating well with those receiving advice and/or care. Ajemain (1993) has summarized the characteristics of effective teams and concluded that being part of an effective team is fun, with members enjoying a sense of belonging and camaraderie. Team members learn to share and interact for the sake of the whole team rather than individual aspirations, thereby giving a structure to the dynamics between team members. Vulnerabilities as well as strengths need to be commonly shared, with difficulties between team members being addressed face to face. This personal exchange can lead to professional growth. None of these things just happens overnight. It takes time and a degree of self-examination to know how you are reacting and relating to team members.

Team reviews should also include social gatherings. Pub lunches, picnics, theatre visits, and other outings are relaxing and therapeutic. They stop reviews from becoming sombre and introspective. Team members, particularly new ones, find that it is much easier in these situations to establish relationships with each other, particularly if there are lingering memories about the person who occupied the post previously.

Reviews can also be useful for reflecting on deaths which have been particularly difficult. Attempts should be made to define 'what' and 'who' contributed to the stressful death. If possible, alternative strategies should be defined to prevent similar problems happening again.

Leadership

Team leadership is a complex task. How this task is fulfilled will often vary depending on the team composition.

There are many approaches to leadership theory (Johnson and Johnson 1975) the main three being:

- the *position approach* where a person is given authority to lead
- the *style approach* incorporating autocracy, democracy, and laissez-faire (Lewin *et al.* 1939)
- the *distributed function* approach where tasks of leadership are distributed throughout the group.

Within the context of palliative care teams there is no one leadership approach that is necessarily correct. The situation, the different professions of team members, the skill mix, the personalities, and experience of individual team members all necessitate that leadership is a very individual consideration for each team.

Thelen (1965) argues that leadership is a team effort and that the various functions of leadership are never in one person but more often distributed among selected individuals within the total group. The fact that the distributed function approach is described as the most widely practised of all leadership styles (Johnson and Johnson, 1975) bears this out.

The process of leadership has two main roles: a role that is t*ask centred* where attention is on aspects of work and vision, and that of *maintenance* or the socially/emotionally-centred role of leadership that is aware of the needs of those doing the work. It is rare for a single individual to have both these qualities. An arrangement where two people form the basic leadership of a team can be very impressive and not easily destroyed. The 'father' and 'mother' role of the nuclear family has been analogized (Bales 1955) to that of the task and maintenance functions of leadership.

Reflecting on the experiences of setting up and then leading a team has produced the following observations. At the beginning of something totally new there is always a sense of excitement: a pulling together, helping one another, excusing each other's mistakes. Because a small specialist palliative care team comprises highly skilled personnel, a formal management structure can appear out of place. However, someone does need to take the responsibility for leading the team, otherwise a leader will emerge by default. A specialist nurse who has been the instigator of the team and is the only full-time member of the team, may feel it inappropriate to *manage* the doctor or social worker on a team, but what about the other nurse specialist? Just because you are the designated leader, having set up the team and knowing the key hospital personnel, does not necessarily mean you have all the other qualities of leadership. In this situation, the leadership roles can be shared. Some autocratic decisions need to be made in times of 'emergency' but generally democratic decisions are taken with group members feeling free to suggest changes.

A stable team can promote tremendous growth for the team itself and for individual team members. It allows barriers to come down. Problems, even personality issues, can be worked through together. It is important that at least one member of the team takes on the responsibility for noticing the 'ups and downs' of team member's feelings, thereby fulfilling the role of the socio-emotional leader (Bales 1955). This is often a particular skill that can be a natural gift: unfortunately, it is a skill that is often not recognized until the person is no longer around bringing cohesion to the team. It is not necessarily found in the leader of the team.

In order to break the new ground of setting up a team, a high-energy, charismatic leader can be helpful. However, this style can lead to reluctance to hand over responsibilities once the team becomes established. The tendency is to under-develop people rather than encourage a degree of initiative and independence. A high degree of emotional stimulation needs to be tempered. A leader who cares and supports individual group members, who provides meaning and under-standing to situations, has a greater chance of holding a group together and benefiting group members. Of course a team needs vision and clear objectives to work towards but not at the expense of the caring, supportive aspects of leadership.

Team dynamic scenario. . .

Within 18 months of a stable period in the history of a palliative care team, three key people left for career development and other legitimate reasons. One of those team members who left was the doctor. When the team was originally established, the founder and team leader had to be energetic and assertive to get the team accepted. With time, team members developed good, well-worn relationships, both internally and externally. The 'energizer' effect of the early leadership style was not a problem until new members began to join what had been a stable, established team.

The leadership styles required for an evolving group are quite different from those required for an established one. The expectations of the team leader need to change with the appointment of new members. Each new member will come with differing views on leadership. In this example, a reappraisal of the team might have helped the transition. Instead, the instability reactivated the 'energizer' approach. The leader compensated for the lack of transition leadership skills by becoming more involved with the clinical work, feeling the need to excel at least in that area. This was excused subconsciously by the fact that new members on the team were, as yet, not fully confident in their roles and needed time to settle in. There was a desire to protect them from pressure in case they became emotionally exhausted. This meant that less time was available for developing and leading the new group members' potential. What seemed to be a quick answer to the prevailing problem of increased clinical work prevented the ongoing development of the team. The new members of the team had come from strict hierarchical management structures. They found it difficult to fit in with the perceived 'laissez-faire' style of leadership of the 'initial' team. The first reaction of the leader was to feel that the way the team had been led in the past had been wrong. In hindsight the new members may have required a different approach, but this did not negate the other style—it had worked well for those team members at the time. However, at the time the insecurity led to a 'wavering'—being blown about by every whim and fancy. What was it about this group of people that made such a difference? The new doctor on the team was more task focused than the previous doctor and, like the team leader, did not have the previous doctor's specific socio-emotional skills of leadership. By default this role was not fulfilled until the new full-time social worker joined the team. Then, the team was able to restore stability once again.

The duality of task-centred and maintenance-centred roles in leadership is vital for group cohesiveness. The fact that team members fulfil different roles clearly has implications in the appointment of new members. Any skills which facilitate group cohesion that are lost must either be picked up by existing team members or be looked for in potential new members.

Anyone taking on the 'leadership' aspect of teamwork needs to consider the hierarchy in which that leadership is to occur. Leadership does not necessarily mean management. A good leader does not necessarily signify a good manager although it does help. For example, the responsibility for staff appraisals does not need to be vested in the leader. Some teams will do their own appraisals. This could mean the designated 'leader' or the lead nurse or doctor of the team. As the team is built on the multidisciplinary concept, this should not be seen as a backward step. Other teams will organize appraisals outside the team setting, for example nurse specialists being individually appraised by a nurse manager or director of nursing, as well as the clinical director of the directorate in which the team is based.

Fulfilling the educational needs of team members

The emphasis of ongoing education within health care can stretch the resources of a small specialist palliative care team. However, the acquisition of new knowledge and skills is vital.

It is difficult for every member on a palliative care team to be actively involved in educational programmes to further their qualifications. However, team members should support one another by encouraging study leave. As in any team, there has to be give and take. This can cause conflict where different professional bodies are concerned. Being given time off for a postgraduate course may have to substitute for going to other conferences.

The educational needs for those team members not following further postgraduate qualifications is just as great. Attendance at conferences or short courses should be encouraged. Quite apart from a sense of personal growth, more satisfaction will be gained from providing a better service because of the acquired knowledge. It is not sufficient to just increase knowledge when wanting to refine skills; it is necessary to practise skills in a controlled environment. Counselling is an example of a skill that is very important for palliative care team work. There are many practical workshops which are extremely useful. Teaching skills can also be improved in workshop seminars. Mention has already been made of working in a hospice to improve practical skills.

Funding postgraduate courses and conferences can be difficult. Macmillan Cancer Relief, Help the Hospices, pharmaceutical firms, special team funds, and other hospital funds are the main sources by which expenses for conferences are met in the UK.

In some situations an interest to carry out a particular piece of research can coincide with a team member applying to do a higher degree. This is rare but not impossible. Obviously a large project will involve greater funding and personnel commitments. This can be a useful way of 'holding on' to a particular team member while allowing them to expand their potential. It can also bring prestige to the team concerned.

On a smaller scale, it can be helpful for team members to research clinical problems which arise, and then present a short summary to the team. The research and presentation should not be time-consuming, nor relate solely to medical problems. This can be a useful way of improving self-confidence. The traditional model of doctor teaching doctors, nurse teaching nurse, and social worker teaching social worker is thereby broken down. This will further strengthen the team approach.

A sound knowledge of terminal care, and the skills to pass on this knowledge, are essential for the educational role of the palliative team. This role is examined in more detail in the next chapter. The other ways in which the team supports the doctors, nurses, and other hospital staff are also reviewed.

7

Supporting the professional carers

One important aspect of a palliative care team's role is to encourage and support other professional staff in their care for the dying. The needs of ward nurses and doctors have a major impact on the palliative care team. If due attention is not given to this aspect of the work, there is a danger that nursing and medical staff will continue to distance themselves from the terminally ill and ignore their needs, or discharge them prematurely. On the other hand, if the care of the dying is 'taken over' by the palliative care team, who then organize everything themselves without educating and supporting other staff, the ward teams will be de-skilled. Either of these scenarios will cause patient care to suffer. Achieving a balance of clinical involvement, education, and support of ward teams is most likely to improve the overall quality of the dying patient within a hospital setting.

Supporting and meeting the needs of other professional carers is made more difficult when they are not able to acknowledge stress. There are good reasons for this: staff need to suppress intense emotions to maintain a calm demeanour when dealing with emergencies. They have to avoid burdening patients with fears and anxieties. However, these practices have developed into an unwritten code that professionals do not experience stress, or if they do, it is not acceptable to share it with colleagues. Personal pride also plays a part in generating these attitudes—the need to be in control. Past experiences, particularly during training, also strongly support these unwritten codes.

This chapter examines the problems that nurses, doctors, and other health professionals experience when looking after the terminally ill patients. It challenges palliative care teams to extend their support and involvement beyond patients and their families to include the ward teams caring for these patients. Particular attention has been paid to the palliative care team's role in teaching, emphasising the multidisciplinary nature of this work.

Teaching and education

It could be argued that the ultimate aim of a hospital palliative care team is to pass on the skills and philosophy of hospice care so effectively as to 'do itself out of a job'. Although this is an impossible task, especially given the frequency with which hospital staff change and move on, the aim of team members must be to try to pass on skills rather than de-skill ward staff.

Teaching and education of all those involved in caring for the dying are a major feature of the team's role . Traditionally, this teaching is given to nurses and doctors but it is just as important to include occupational therapists, physiotherapists, social workers, and dietitians. Some input should be considered for auxiliary nurses and porters.

Education in palliative care is best delivered in a multidisciplinary way—not just for the teachers but also for the learners. Unfortunately, hospital schedules often prevent this, although it should not deter you when planning more formal study days. Teaching can be carried out both informally and formally. The palliative care team should make sure that both styles of teaching are used.

Informal teaching

Anyone acting as a specialist practitioner must realize that they are potentially 'on show' whenever they are in contact with other people. The clinical involvment clinically at ward level means that most situations can be turned into a teaching opportunity. Junior nurses and doctors can be influenced as they scrutinize team members' attitudes and knowledge. Role-modelling is one of the most useful informal methods of teaching— having the learner come in to see how the expert interacts with the patient or family. This can be carried out across disciplines, for example junior doctors can learn a great deal by accompanying the nurse specialists.

The first visit to see a patient is an ideal time for role modelling. This is when the patient often takes the opportunity to explore what they have been told previously by others. It provides a natural occasion to observe communication techniques and learn how to assess symptoms. You have to work at making these opportunities happen. Ward staff find it difficult to schedule time out of a busy ward routine. It is worth the effort because it will extend the nurse's or doctor's knowledge. It also encourages a closer rapport between the staff and the patient. Sometimes ward staff say that they are too busy to come, because they feel that getting further involved is too costly emotionally. Most staff will make a point in accompanying you because they are keen to extend their knowledge of palliative care. Student nurses or nurses undertaking a specific course on the ward are often very pleased to be involved in this way.

Medical learning is often based on experience gained on the job. Junior doctors quickly become aware that the preferences of their seniors take precedence over any prior formal teaching. When faced with a patient complaining of pain or some other distressing symptom, the doctor may occasionally ask the nurses for advice. Usually, they will refer to the senior registrar or consultant, whose advice will become the basis for future decisions. This is one reason why myths about the use of morphine are perpetuated .

The palliative care team should exploit the importance of experiential learning. Whenever the team recommends a change in a patient's management, they should discuss the reasoning with the house staff, preferably in person rather than by phone. The policy of the palliative care team doctor not writing prescriptions means junior hospital staff are more likely to become proficient with the use of drugs such as morphine. The majority of the junior doctors will be grateful for this support. They will then want to phone or talk about other patients who do not necessarily need to be seen by the team.

In more practical situations, the palliative care team member should supervise rather than carry out the procedure themselves. Examples include setting up syringe pumps to administer subcutaneous opioids, or re-dressing and changing epidural syringes. This should ensure that the palliative care team is not seen as the sole repository of experience and knowledge about terminal care.

Ward rounds can be an important place for sharing knowledge, both about the physical control of symptoms as well as psychosocial care. Discussions during ward rounds often touch on ethical dilemmas, and team members should feel able to debate important issues. It can be very daunting to speak at some meetings, especially in a high powered oncology talk-round. Even if you cannot contribute very much in the beginning it is worthwhile persevering, especially if one has been invited to attend. You will become more confident with time, and will learn from the meetings meanwhile.

Recently, the transfer of nurse education to colleges or universities has left little opportunity for the palliative care team members to be involved in their teaching at classroom level. This makes informal teaching at ward level even more important. Small, low-key 'teach-ins' on the ward are a further ideal format for informal teaching. However, there is less 'overlap' of nurses shifts in the afternoon, which makes this more difficult to organize. These sessions can be tailored to specific problems on the ward, or to requests for certain topics. If numbers on one ward are low, to make it worthwhile the session can usefully be shared with another ward or floor.

Formal teaching

Formal teaching should be a feature of a hospital palliative care team, although it is not always easy to schedule. The very nature of the team's clinical work is quite unpredictable. Sometimes there are only a few new referrals to see one week; then there are more than can be coped with the next. Inevitably it works out that the very week you have scheduled a couple of workshops or a study day, the team is inundated with new referrals to see. This can be very taxing but should not dampen the enthusiasm for education!

Lectures, workshops, study days, and involvement in orientation programmes need to be properly planned as part of the teaching structure. As long as you do not plan too much for one week without taking into consideration annual leave and other scheduled meetings, generally it will work well. You will soon realize the mistake of planning too many fixed meetings in a week. Unfortunately the best planned teaching schedule does not necessarily secure attendance—there are so many other influences that can frustrate a teaching programme.

There is a considerable amount of formal teaching that can be done, especially at a university or teaching hospital. It is vital to speak to organizers of in-service training for nurses or the undergraduate programme for junior doctors to ensure you are included in the general programmes. Formal lectures may be difficult to fit into already crowded medical student curricula. The number of lectures will depend on the commitment of the coordinators of the teaching programme. Teaching for medical students and doctors is usually carried out by the doctor on the team but it is valuable to use the clinical nurse specialist, social worker, and chaplain to promote the multidisciplinary approach.

Most medical students and junior doctors are keen to learn something about the treatment of pain, nausea, and vomiting because these problems also occur in patients who are not terminally ill. In the UK, palliative care is a specialty in its own right. Medical colleges have begun to include palliative care teaching into various modules of the curriculum, especially in the community and psychiatry modules. Learning is improved if students are examined on the basics of pain relief, particularly the use of morphine. In the ward setting, the palliative care team worker should discuss any patients with the medical students who are assigned to them. Students may appreciate accompanying the key worker when their patient is seen. This will supplement their theoretical experience. Some medical students want to spend time with the palliative care team: either short visits for one or two days, or longer periods as part of an elective.

Some teams and medical colleges organize small group sessions to help improve communication. The use of role play and video recordings of mock interviews help to prepare students for the difficult job of breaking bad news. The specialist registrar or consultant in palliative medicine who has an interest in communication issues can not only highlight listening and communication skills but also promote the care of the dying and the palliative care team. Exposing students to dramatic emotional reactions in a controlled situation is often helpful (Hoy *et al.* 1984) in preparing them for real life situations. These methods can be extended to include junior doctors and members of other disciplines (Nash 1984).

A useful workshop has been the 'Breaking Bad News' breakfast. Coffee and croissants (always a good incentive) were provided by the department requesting the workshop. Members from the palliative care team would start the discussion. Informal conversation about the difficulties of breaking bad news, and various scenarios would then be shared by those present. For doctors, the beginning of the day can be quite a good time for teaching. The breakfasts were well attended (including the consultants) and acted as a support as well as a teaching session. Such workshops are particularly helpful for junior doctors and can be held 2–3 times at the beginning of either the house officer or senior house officer rotations. Another alternative is to use drug company sponsorship for a lunch. This can be an important opportunity to update professionals on new drugs for pain and symptom control.

The multidisciplinary role of the palliative care team should be exploited in teaching. However, there are definitely occasions when it is more appropriate for the nurse specialists to be teaching the nurses and for the doctor on the team to be teaching the junior doctors. Throughout their training junior doctors are scheduled specific teaching on each specialty they are attached to. Getting included on these sessions can be very useful, for example teaching pain and symptom control on the oncology rotation.

When planning the content of formal lectures for nurses, it is important to be aware of their perceived needs. These needs vary considerably with length of experience and seniority (Hockley 1989). By the end of their final year in training, many student nurses can talk to patients without feeling self-conscious. They become more aware of the needs of families and want to learn about coping with the relatives' questions and emotions. The fundamentals of symptom control can be intermingled with teaching on psychodynamics.

The unpredictability of ward work can make on-going education frustrating because of the low attendance. Some teams have found that organizing 'rolling workshops' can overcome these difficulties. Here the same subject is repeated so that nurses on different shifts can get a chance to attend. In one hospital all the nurse specialists respresenting the different areas take a particular afternoon a week and run a programme over a 6–10 week period. The programme is then repeated as rolling workshops. The palliative care representation in these workshops is very important. For more specific ward or directorate teaching, tutorials can be taped so that nurses on different shifts or even on night duty can listen to the tapes and keep their knowledge up to date.

It is much less common to be involved in formal teaching at consultant level. However, the opportunity to give presentations at medical and surgical grand rounds can provide a platform for reviewing issues such as the management of neurogenic pain, or making difficult ethical decisions.

The theory of teaching different disciplines at the same time is a wonderful idea but very difficult to achieve in reality. It is near impossible to finding suitable times when nurses and doctors can come together. Despite these problems, it is important to try to organize at least one local multidisciplinary palliative conference on palliative care in the acute setting every 1–2 years.

Inevitably, team members are asked to take part in more and more lectures or study days. Some way of monitoring and controlling requests will be necessary, otherwise clinical involvement will suffer. It is wise for a palliative care team to set limits for education, just as a team may have to limit the number of new referrals. One of the boundaries may well be no lectures outside the hospital, or no more than two lecture visits outside the city per month. When responding to invitations to speak at symposia, thought needs to be given to the availability of resources on the team.

Written guidelines (pain, nausea and vomiting, constipation) and booklets (bereavement, palliative care drug lists in the hospital formulary) are another method of influencing care. They provide a good basis for carrying out audit. Research shows that the writing of guidelines is most beneficial for those people who actually write them. It is therefore important to include staff who will be involved in putting them into practice, for example ward staff and pharmacy. Working with people on creating guidelines and booklets helps promote the team as well as advance knowledge.

Support

The support needed by ward nurses and doctors working with terminally ill patients will vary from ward to ward and from hospital to hospital. The type of support for a ward team will depend on the attitude, leadership, and expertise of the ward sister, senior doctors, and management.

Nurses are more exposed to the needs and difficulties of the dying than other health professionals. This is because they are with the patient more often. Many of the support issues discussed in this section are aimed at nurses. Ward teams which learn to communicate and work well together as a multidisciplinary team will manifest less stress. Palliative care teams must be alert to and build on these strengths whenever possible.

Professional stressors

When student nurses start training in hospitals, they have usually never had experience of coping with death. Within a few weeks, they are often caring for patients who die. Whitfield (1979) found this was one of their most stressful experiences. By contrast, medical students have much less exposure to the terminally ill. Up to 30% of medical students graduate without ever having had to manage a dying patient (Ahmedzai 1982). Medical training makes it harder for doctors to acknowledge stress beyond a relatively intimate group of peers. Medical students have to develop a toughened exterior to withstand a teaching programme which does not allow the student to say 'I do not know'. As doctors progresses into postgraduate training, even peer support tends to subside. The pressure to maintain a smooth unruffled professional appearance becomes greater (McCue 1982).

Because health professionals often find it difficult to recognize and deal with stress, they may present patients and families as problems for the palliative care team. The true situation becomes apparent when the patient denies being distressed by or even having the symptoms that were recorded in the referrals. The ward staff will resist and may even resent any effort by the palliative care team to shift the focus back onto them.

When a student nurse feels under stress, the busy nature of acute wards, coupled with the vulnerability of senior staff to the same stresses, makes it difficult to get support. Newly trained nurses experience stress when left in charge of wards where patients are dying. Primary nursing or team nursing requires quite junior trained nurses to take greater responsibility for patient care. Newly trained nurses may not have the skills and experience needed to deal with the different situations faced in caring for the dying, particularly the young dying. This is not a problem if the ward leader is very experienced. However, if they are also less experienced then nurses may have more responsibility put upon them than is emotionally sustainable.

In these scenarios, palliative care team members must try to make time not only to help the individual nurse but also to support the whole team, especially if there are complicated medical problems. Occasionally, the stress may be so severe that the ward team cannot follow the advice of the palliative care team Considerable patience is required, rising above the frustration that is felt when advice is declined. This is sometimes difficult if the palliative care team is having to cope with a lot of other pressing work. Other palliative care team members need to be aware of the dilemma and be prepared to take on some of the other work. This will free up the time needed to deal with the complex ward situation. If there are no other team members to fulfil this role, it may be necessary to cancel meetings to give one the necessary space.

The on-going reduction in the number of nurses working on wards is very stressful for ward teams. Nursing procedures are more difficult to carry out and this contributes to high rates of staff turnover. The palliative care team cannot directly influence these factors; indeed the ward staff can become jealous of the time that the team members have to sit and talk with patients, only then to give advice and not help with practical care. Helping with procedures may be a valuable public relations exercise when a ward is very busy. It is also helpful to talk about and acknowledge the difficulties that ward staff are experiencing, even though you may be powerless to bring about any change. The fact that some one appreciates the problems will contrast with the administration who continually expect that standards of care be maintained despite reduced staff numbers.

When a ward is not busy, it is important to spend short periods of time socializing, perhaps chatting informally over a cup of tea. This will serve to monitor the emotional state of the wards. By getting to know the nurses and ward clerks before crises develop, you can identify who might be at risk from stress. It will also help the nurses feel less threatened when you come to discuss difficulties.

Patient and family related stressors

The majority of nurses find performing good nursing care rewarding. It is frequently identified as a major reason for entering the profession. They identify their prime aim in caring for the terminally ill as keeping the patient as pain free and comfortable as possible. Practical procedures such as dealing with incontinence and vomiting, dressing offensive wounds, and feeding the patient are generally not stressful. However, dealing with certain symptoms such as pain, breathlessness, and the 'death rattle' are distressing (Hockley 1989). Clearly, the palliative care team can reduce this distress by improving patients' symptoms, and educating the nurses about the principles of symptom control. However, the stress of the nurses will be increased if re-education of the doctors is not an integral part of the team's teaching role.

The psychological needs of the patient and family are frequently rated as distressing. Anxious patients, or patients who ask questions about whether they are dying, cause as much stress as uncontrolled physical symptoms. Difficulties arise with young patients; nurses may identify with the patient and young family. Aggressive patients may arouse anger and frustration, and, at the same time, a sense of guilt; negative feelings are considered inappropriate for professional carers.

Doctors may have difficulty dealing with patients with advanced cancer. Disease relapse and death are seen as failures now that technological innovations can prolong life. The need for a sense of accomplishment, coupled with a desire to protect patients from distress, will motivate doctors to take credit for 'curing' cancer with an operation or some other treatment. Buckman (1984) noted that ward rounds and clinics proceed more smoothly and quickly if the probability of future relapse is glossed over with phrases such as 'we have got it in time'. He then describes the patient's anger and anxiety when the disease relapses. Primary teams often refer patients to the palliative care team when this happens. It is helpful to involve the primary team in dealing with the symptoms and other problems. You can reduce the sense of failure by encouraging participation, and offering several treatment strategies. When the patient improves, the staff share in the sense of satisfaction. They become more positive with future patients who cannot be cured. Rarely, some doctors prefer to opt out altogether, and the palliative care team virtually takes over.

Cancer patients with previous psychological difficulties may be branded as 'problem' patients. Pain and other symptoms tend to be re-labelled as anxiety. These patients will frequently be referred to the palliative care team, even by staff who will not use the team for difficult symptom control problems. It is surprising how often the primary team becomes more responsive to the patient when the palliative care team diverts 'problem' behaviours away from the doctors by paying attention to the patient's needs.

The stress of caring for relatives reflects, in part, the tendency for families to displace anxiety and even anticipatory grief on to the ward staff. It is compounded by the fact that at least 50% of relatives of dying patients may not see any doctors during their loved one's final admission (Hockley *et al.* 1988). Even when the patient is relatively well, doctors often fail to convey the reasoning behind important treatment decisions. If nurses feel unable to relay this information, tension can arise between families and the ward team. These tensions may affect relationships within the ward team itself. Even when patients and families are told, they often do not ask questions at the time. Subsequently, the nursing staff may have to bear the brunt of the criticisms and questions

On occasions, genuine time pressures will make doctors curtail interviews or prevent them picking up the patient cues which herald questions. The extra time available to the palliative care team is helpful. By reviewing patients before clinics or ward rounds, medical problems can be selected out and presented to the doctors. The more time-consuming psychosocial problems can subsequently be dealt with by the team member. It may also be helpful for the palliative care team doctor to prescribe medications for urgent symptom control when the doctors on the primary team are in the operating theatre or casualty.

Occasionally, pressure of time is used to cover up uncertainty and lack of experience. Uncertainty may relate to not knowing how to initiate an interview, or how to deal with the ensuing emotional reactions. The family may fuel the doctor's fear that sharing bad news will cause the patient to 'give up' or be distressed. It is often easier to give the family more information about the illness and prognosis. The palliative care team can break down these barriers by indicating when the patient wants to talk about prognosis, and then give advice about the response. The temptation is always to respond immediately and directly. This may be appropriate on occasions. However, taking up the patient's questions with the primary firm will give them more confidence. It will also enhance the rapport between the palliative care team and the patient.

Making treatment decisions about patients with advanced cancer or other life-threatening illnesses can be a major source of stress (Degner and Beaton 1987). The emphasis on teaching the basic sciences at medical college leaves doctors ill-prepared for the uncertainty of clinical practice. Decisions frequently have to be made on the basis of conflicting or incomplete information. A decision for treatment may involve exposing the patients to considerable risk for marginal benefits. Financial and legal constraints play an increasing role in the decision-making process.

Patients and families are becoming increasingly less satisfied with a passive role in the decision-making process. Patients may want to push for treatments that are unacceptable to the primary team. If the primary team accedes, they worry about the risk of toxicity or death; if they decline, there is the risk of patient anger. The primary team will often appreciate your confirmation of their decision to proceed ahead with the patient's wish. However, if the primary team do not support the patient's view, it may be possible to gently voice an alternative opinion. This can be useful if you have a good rapport with the specific team, even if the opinion is not heeded. It serves as a reminder that excellent medical care does not always require active treatments. The importance of the palliative care team being familiar with the theoretical basis for decision-making is emphasized in chapter 5.

A dying patient may upset other patients nearby, which can cause stress for the staff. Neighbouring patients are often not told when a terminally ill patient dies; they are usually left to guess. Occasionally they may even be told something else, for example that the deceased has been transferred to another hospital. The other nurses then face the added stress of participating in a collusion, fearing that their relationship with these patients will be undermined.

Palliative care team members should feel comfortable dealing with these situations, particularly if they have trained in a hospice. However, they must resist the tendency to take over from the ward staff. Although stress levels will be reduced if the team intervenes, the nurses may not learn by the experience. They will become more reliant on the palliative care team. The ward staff, particularly the patient's primary nurse, should be encouraged to accompany the palliative care team member when the patient is seen. Observing, and hopefully participating will improve nurses' confidence. When the nurse manages similar psychological problems in the future, this effort should be recognized by the palliative care team and given due praise.

Rarely, there will be difficult situations when symptoms cannot be controlled or psychosocial problems resolved. The palliative care team may feel the same sense of failure and stress as the primary team. The palliative care team must continue to support the nursing staff just as they continue to visit the patient and family. The doctors and nurses should not be abandoned because they have to continue caring. Even if nothing more is possible, staying involved in the situation will help. Sharing your frustrations and sense of inadequacy in a controlled way will encourage them to accept their feelings.

Support groups

The use of regular support groups for staff has been widely debated in the palliative care literature. Although they are more commonly used by hospices, support groups have been extremely useful in some oncology units. How often and who actually directs such a group will vary. If the palliative care team do not initiate, and it is often best that the idea comes from ward staff themselves, then these groups are often set up by concerned ward sisters. However, they are best led by a psychologist, specialist social worker, or interested chaplain. The groups need to be held regularly—every 2 to 4 weeks.

Support groups are particularly important on wards where there are frequent deaths. However, finding a right time for everyone is never easy and it requires commited staff to organize them. Over a lunchtime is one idea, but then there is the difficulty of having to go back into the clinical setting after a session of sharing deep emotions. If the group is run well then staff will want to use it whatever the time, because of the benefits they feel. The group should include the whole ward team, not only the nurses and doctors but also ward clerks and even the cleaners as appropriate.

It is always very difficult to know how to structure these meetings. Nothing is worse than a group sitting round gazing at the floor feeling that they are just coming to make up the numbers. There has to be a purpose. One structure is to discuss the deaths that have occurred during the weeks since the last meeting. Staff can rate the different aspects of care by giving a score out of 10 which can then open up discussion. This provides a safe starting point, which can then lead into discussions about how the death affected the staff. These group meetings can be interspersed with teach-ins and videos on issues like grief or team dynamics.

In some ward situations it is inappropriate to run a regular support group. There may not be the right people to run a group, or there may not be enough deaths on a ward to warrant one. Nonetheless, it is still important to try to meet with staff after a particularly difficult death or after a number of deaths in rapid succession. If there were difficult pain problems or complex medical issues then the junior doctors on the ward should be encouraged to attend. Choosing the right time when everyone can be present is nearly impossible. However, the meeting should not occur too soon after the death. To wait a few days to allow emotions and tensions to settle can help to diffuse any feelings of animosity and enables a more supportive session to take place.

The sessions should not be didactic in nature; everyone should be encouraged to share their experiences. This provides an opportunity to share feelings about difficulties and to identify topics for further discussion and education. Staff confidence can be restored by acknowledging aspects of care that were done well.

Multidisciplinary stressors and support

There is no doubt that different problems associated with caring for the dying cause differing degrees of stress to different professionals. One of the strengths of hospice philosophy has been the emphasis on the multi-disciplinary approach to care. When members on the palliative care team are seen supporting each other and relating across the professions, ward teams will be encouraged to do the same.

A common interdisciplinary issue arises when nurses disagree with the prescription of a treatment. This places them in conflict with the doctors. The difficulty arises because patients often share their deepest fears and anxieties about the medical management with the nurses. At times, nurses misinterpret what the patient is saying: 'I do not like treatment' is not the same as 'I do not want treatment'. Sometimes nurses project their own fears about treatment on to the patients. In these situations, it is important for the palliative care team to clarify what the patient is really saying and help the nurses to support the patient's choice. However, when the nurse is in tune with the wishes of the patient the palliative care team should assist in taking up the issues with the medical team.

When it is not possible to change the attitudes or decisions of the medical team, it will still be important to confirm that the nurses are correct in their interpretation. This helps the nursing staff maintain their sense of personal worth and ability, which are so often undermined when nurses' perceptions are at variance with those of the doctors—'the doctors must be right'. Relaying the doctors' perceptions of the problem and reasoning for decisions, if these can be identified, may be valuable. It is usually very difficult to facilitate a situation of open dialogue.

The nursing staff are very quick usually to realize the palliative care team's potential for reducing stress. They will often want to refer terminally ill patients before the doctors do. If the team accepts referrals from nurses, there is a risk of exacerbating stress should the doctors take exception. As stated earlier it is wise to check that the senior doctors of the ward team would like specialist palliative care advice. Asking the nurse to go back and check with the doctors will also encourage multidisciplinary collaboration within the ward team.

The continual turnover of junior house staff may cause difficulties, especially because they are usually responsible for prescribing the medications necessary for symptom control. Patient care suffers when the doctor is not familiar with drugs like morphine and ward nurses are not confident about dosages when asked for guidance. The stress of educating each new set of house staff is made easier by involving the palliative care team. Some allowance for an increase in referrals during the induction of new house staff can be useful.

Paramedical staff such as occupational therapists, physiotherapists, and dietitians often complain that their skills are often undervalued and under-utilized. Terminally ill patients frequently benefit from their expertise. However, these staff may be unaware of the special needs of terminally ill patients, especially the sense of urgency required when patients are deteriorating quickly. The palliative care team should make a special point of discussing relevant problems with these staff . The opportunity to share information will enhance their enthusiasm and satisfaction, as well as patient care. It might be appropriate to invite particular paramedical staff and chaplains to the team's weekly multidisciplinary meeting especially if there are complex situations to discuss.

Pharmacists who work in the acute hospital setting now have a higher profile on the wards and in various departments. Their recommendations can occasionally undermine information given by nurse specialists. Pharmacists have greater theoretical knowledge of drug therapy but less clinical experience in uncovering the cause of the symptom. Greater clinical teamwork can be achieved by collaborating with interested pharmacists on various guidelines. Nurse specialists use their knowledge of medications alongside their clinical evaluation of the patient. Every opportunity should be taken to discuss alternative drugs, routes of administration, or costings.

The needs of other health professionals should be considered by the palliative care team. It is important to get to know the ward clerks. They frequently have to cope with staff stress, as well as handle their own sense of loss when patients die. Medical typists, out-patient clerks, radiographers, laboratory, and other staff will appreciate a personal approach when you want to expedite an appointment or results. Always remember to thank them for their help. This contrasts sharply with the usual impersonal telephone calls they receive.

Palliative care teams frequently relate to different specialties at ward level. It is not unusual, however, to find yourself entwined between inter-professional opinions. This is most likely to occur when the team is asked to see a patient on a surgical or medical ward at the same time as the oncologist or radiotherapist. It may be best to wait until the other teams have clarified their decisions before you rush in to see the patient or family. There will be times, for example, when a surgeon's decision to ask for an oncologist's opinion will mean that the oncologist may not want the palliative care team involved. Your approach to interdisciplinary decision-making will change with time as the different disciplines feel more comfortable with your role. It helps if the team doctor is able to maintain a consistently high profile at ward level.

There are three services that a palliative care team may be specifically involved with:

• the pain clinic
• radiotherapy
• medical oncology.

The next chapter reviews the contribution of these services to the care of patients with advanced cancer.

8

The pain clinic and palliative oncology

The pain clinic and oncology services have an important role in treating pain and other symptoms of advanced cancer. Obviously, the role of the palliative care team will overlap with these services. There is the potential for misunderstanding and conflict; although such services may feel threatened by a palliative care team, the problem is not one-sided. If palliative care team members have not worked in a pain clinic or oncology ward, they may be ignorant of the benefits these services can offer. These team members may want to 'protect' patients from 'aggressive' treatments, and only use symptomatic medical treatment.

To help overcome these problems, we have reviewed the roles of the pain clinic and oncology services. We have provided insights about how oncologists decide to treat patients, and guidelines for working with oncology services.

The pain clinic

Role of the pain clinic in the management of cancer pain

The commonest symptom experienced by patients with advanced cancer is pain. It has been estimated that in 90% of these patients, satisfactory pain control can be obtained by pharmacological means alone. In the remaining 10%, however, referral to a pain clinic for specialized techniques for the relief of pain may be required. This latter figure may be an underestimate. At one hospice which was visited weekly by a pain clinic anaesthetist, 22.7% of the patients admitted underwent a specialized pain-relieving procedure (Saunders 1986). This emphasizes the need for palliative care teams to establish and maintain close links with a pain clinic or an anaesthetist with a special interest in nerve blocks.

General principles

The assessment of the patient's pain, its cause, and the patient's reaction to it are an important function of the pain clinic and an essential preliminary to successful management. In particular, the location, characteristics, and temporal factors of the pain must be noted and a full neurological examination of the relevant area documented. If possible, the examiner should try to distinguish between local peripheral pain and referred pain, and between somatic and autonomic pain, as well as documenting which nerve or nerves are involved. The anticipated procedure and any potential complications must be discussed with the patient, the referring medical and nursing staff, and, if possible, the patients' relatives.

Before embarking on a permanent nerve block it is advisable, if practicable, to perform a diagnostic local anaesthetic block to enable both the patient to experience the likely benefits of a permanent block and the doctor to confirm the accuracy of the diagnosis (Foster 1990).

Available techniques

Specialized techniques for the relief of pain can be classified into the following two groups:

- Techniques which interrupt the pain pathway. The pain pathway can be interrupted peripherally (i.e. with a nerve block) or centrally. These techniques are the most commonly used for the control of cancer pain.
- Techniques which relieve pain by stimulation of the peripheral and central nervous systems (e.g. acupuncture, transcutaneous nerve stimulation, and implanted stimulators) (Foster 1990).

Nerve blocks

The commonest indications for a nerve block are:

- localized pain breaking through otherwise adequate analgesia
- pain controlled at rest, but not on movement
- attempt to reduce analgesic dose (to reduce the side-effects of systemic analgesics)
- failure of systemic analgesics to control pain.

Methods used for nerve blocks

The pain can be interrupted by the following methods:

- Local anaesthetic agents: the commonest agents used are lignocaine, bupivacaine, prilocaine, and ropivacaine.
- Neurolytic agents: phenol and alcohol are the most frequently used. The great advantage of this method is that a minimum of equipment is required and, in many instances, they are an adequate substitute for major neurosurgical procedures. However, these chemicals destroy nerve fibres indiscriminately, and therefore accurate and discrete placement of the agent is essential.
- Cryolesion: the cryoprobe produces an ice ball at the probe tip. The nerve is placed within the ice ball and repeated freeze–thaw cycles cause wallerian degeneration and axonal disruption. This technique causes fewer complications than neurolytic agents, but the duration of analgesia is very variable, from a few days to several months.
- Radiofrequency thermocoagulation: with the aid of a stimulating current, an electrode is accurately localized to the appropriate nerve. By means of a high-frequency electrical current, thermocoagulation of the nerve elements occurs. This technique has the advantage of a low incidence of complications and is superseding the use of neurolytic agents on peripheral nerves. The procedure does, however, require considerable expertise and the equipment is expensive.
- Spinal opiates: the discovery of opiate receptors in the spinal cord has led to the extensive use of spinal opioids by both subarachnoid and epidural routes. Nausea and vomiting, pruritus, urinary retention, and respiratory depression have all been reported but these side-effects and complications are usually self-limiting and can be managed by adjusting the opioid dose (Cousins *et al.* 1988). Long-term use of spinal opioid administration involves either a percutaneous catheter or a totally implantable system. Infection is the predominant complication.

Combinations of local anaesthetics and spinal opioids produce analgesia for pains poorly responsive to opioids alone and can be particularly useful for neuropathic cancer pain. Other non-opioid agents which have been used by the spinal route include clonidine, an alpha2-adrenergic agonist, and baclofen, a GABA receptor agonist.

Spinal neurolysis

In general, spinal neurolysis is best reserved for patients with advanced cancer and well localized pain limited to a few spinal segments. The spinal nerve can be blocked at the different sites:

- Subarachnoid neurolysis: the injection of a neurolytic agent onto a spinal nerve requires few special facilities and equipment, and this technique can be made widely available. Useful analgesia is experienced in 70% of cases. The most serious complications are motor paresis and interference with bladder and rectal sphincters. Subarachnoid neurolysis is most commonly used for bilateral saddle pain and localized pain in the trunk.
- Epidural neurolysis: this theoretically offers the advantage of fewer complications than the subarachnoid route, but the analgesia is not usually as effective. The commonest indication is thoracic and upper abdominal pain.
- Subdural neurolysis: this procedure can be particularly useful for treating pain in the distribution of the cervical nerve roots, but the technique is complex and requires x-ray facilities (Lipton 1979).

Peripheral nerve blocks

In general, peripheral nerve blockade produces relatively short-lived pain relief, as compared with spinal neurolysis. Radiofrequency thermocoagulation of peripheral nerves is, however, more effective than peripheral chemical neurolysis or cryoanalgesia. Peripheral nerve blocks are most commonly used for pain in the head and neck, thorax, and brachial plexus. Local anaesthetics, if given by a continuous infusion via a catheter, can be particularly useful and the recently described technique of interpleural analgesia has been modified for upper abdominal and thoracic cancer pain (Fineman 1989)

Autonomic blocks

There are many instances in which some or all of the cancer pain is due to involvement of autonomic nerves and for which block of this system is indicated.

The most commonly used autonomic blocks are:

- Stellate ganglion block: the stellate ganglion supplies the head, neck upper limbs, and thorax. Tumour spread in the upper thorax sometimes involves sympathetic fibres causing oedema, cyanosis, and a burning pain in the arm. In such cases, a stellate ganglion block will be valuable. Other conditions where consideration should be given are in scar pain following a radical mastectomy and in Pancoast's tumour (Foster 1990).

- Coeliac plexus block: the coeliac plexus supplies the upper abdominal viscera. Coeliac plexus block produces prolonged relief of upper abdominal and back pain in over 80% of patients with pancreatic and gastric cancer (Saltzburg and Foley 1989). The splanchnic nerve block (Boas 1983) may be a safer alternative to the coeliac plexus block.
- Lumbar sympathetic block: the lumbar sympathetic chain supplies pelvic and urogenital viscera and the lower limbs. Pain from carcinoma of rectum, bladder, and uterus may be helped by lumbar sympathetic blockade (Bristow and Foster 1988). Some patients with tumours in the pelvis develop burning pain in the lower limb, and this can be relieved by lumbar sympathetic blockade.
- Superior hypogastric plexus block: this has recently been described in the management of pelvic cancer pain (Plancarte *et al.* 1990a). This block may be more selective for pelvic pain than lumbar sympathetic block.
- Ganglion of Walther (ganglion Impar) block: this is a useful technique for perineal pain with a low risk of complications (Plancarte *et al.* 1990b).

Upper limb
Peripheral nerve blockade of the upper limbs is complicated by a high risk to motor function. However, brachial plexus neurolysis should be considered in patients with carcinomatous involvement of the brachial plexus, Pancoast's tumour, and pathological fractures of the upper limb (Charlton 1986). Subdural neurolytic blocks can be very useful for shoulder pain. However, the analgesia is often short-lived and the technique is complex. Some arm pain may have both a sympathetic and somatic component, and sympathetic blockade by stellate ganglion block may be of benefit (see above).

Lower limb
Subarachnoid block is the most useful nerve block for pain in the lumbosacral root distribution, with an overall success rate of over 70%. The complications of motor paresis and bladder and rectal dysfunction can be kept to less than 2% by careful selection of patients and scrupulous attention to technique. The regional hip block, performed by local anaesthetic blockade of the obturator nerve and nerve to quadratus

femoris (Lipton 1979), can last several months in patients with acetabular or femoral lesions. This procedure carries virtually no risks. Lumbar sympathetic blockade should always be considered for patients with burning pain and hyperpathia in the lower limb (see above).

Head and neck

The most commonly performed peripheral nerve block in the head and neck is of the trigeminal ganglion, and this block can be useful for the control of pain from advanced orofacial malignancy. Block of the whole trigeminal nerve may not be necessary as orofacial malignancies usually involve only the lower two divisions and the maxillary and mandibular nerves are amenable to nerve blockade.

Glossopharyngeal and vagus nerve blocks may be needed when pain is arising from the pharynx, larynx, and related structures, and subdural neurolysis is useful for pain in the distribution of the cervical roots.

Thorax

Paravertebral and intercostal nerve blocks are useful for pain due to small metastases, pathological rib fractures, and breast cancer. However, these peripheral nerve blocks are most effective if limited to no more than 2–3 roots. More widespread pain is better managed by epidural neurolysis, spinal opiates, or interpleural analgesia.

Abdomen and pelvis

Coeliac plexus block can relieve pain in over 80% of patients with pancreatic and gastric cancer, and patients should undergo this block as soon as conventional analgesics are inadequate. Splanchnic nerve block is an alternative procedure.

Pelvic visceral pain due to rectal, bladder, or uterine cancer is often relieved by lumbar sympathetic or superior hypogastric block. Widespread abdominal and pelvic pain is best managed by spinal opioids.

Perineal pain is relieved by subarachnoid (intrathecal) neurolytic block, although this procedure carries some risk to bladder and rectal function. Useful alternatives to subarachnoid neurolysis, such as transsacral nerve block, ganglion of Walther block, and caudal epidural cryolesion have been described but, although the risks to sphincter function with these techniques is negligible, pain relief by these methods is usually of short duration.

Cordotomy

Cordotomy is the most common central method used for interrupting the pain pathway. The anterolateral quadrant of the spinal cord can be sectioned surgically (open cordotomy) or, more commonly nowadays, percutaneously with a radiofrequency probe (percutaneous cervical cordotomy). Cordotomy should be considered for:

- unilateral cancer pain
- pain below C5 dermatome
- pain of well-defined dermatomal distribution
- short life expectancy.

The main complication of a cordotomy is motor weakness in the ipsilateral lower limb; 20% of patients experience difficulty in walking after the procedure. However, over 80% of patients obtain total relief of unilateral pain following a percutaneous cervical cordotomy (Lipton 1979).

Pituitary ablation

A trans-sphenoidal approach to the pituitary gland is made and the gland is destroyed either with a small volume of alcohol or by the application of a cryoprobe.

This technique is particularly useful for diffuse pain due to widespread bony metastases from hormone-dependent tumours (breast, prostate, kidney, thyroid), but has also been used, empirically, with success for non-hormone-dependent malignant pain when other methods have failed or are unavailable. The mechanism of action is unknown. Of patients with a hormone-dependent tumour, 70% are relieved of their pain but the procedure does carry a mortality of 5%, and most patients develop diabetes insipidus (Lipton 1979).

Stimulation techniques

Some documented evidence exists on the use of acupuncture in cancer pain, one study demonstrating that 56% of patients gained improvement for 7 days (Filshie 1990). The use of transcutaneous nerve stimulation in cancer pain shows a wide range of efficacy (15–99%), which may be due to the many variables involved (Ostrowski 1979).

Some good results have been report with spinal cord stimulation, but it is generally believed that spinal cord stimulation is not a good first choice for patients with cancer pain unless there is a signifcant component of neuropathic pain in the pain syndrome (Meyerson 1990).

Hypnosis

Although hypnosis has been used in some units with varying degrees of success (Spiegel 1985), it would seem unlikely that this technique will replace more conventional methods of treating malignant pain.

Non-cancer pain

Patients with cancer are as likely as the remainder of the population to suffer from non-cancer pain. Referral of a patient suffering from cancer to a pain clinic for advice and management of non-malignant pain may be appropriate.

Palliative oncology

In general, radiotherapy and chemotherapy are administered in designated cancer centres and units (Calman and Hine 1995). Occasionally, hormone therapy and less toxic chemotherapy may be prescribed by surgeons and physicians on general wards. A significant percentage of cancer patients will be considered for these treatments. It therefore behoves palliative care teams to be aware of the principles and practice of anti-cancer treatment, particularly if working in a cancer centre. Even in hospitals without such services, you may become involved with patients who would be appropriate for referral, or be asked to provide local follow-up for patients on active treatment elsewhere.

We have not tried to provide an in-depth description of these treatment modalities, and there is considerable variation in the practice thereof from unit to unit. Nevertheless, some basic concepts will be outlined which will facilitate shared care, particularly if you have not had previous oncology experience.

The first important concept is the meaning of the word 'palliative'. In the hospice setting, 'palliative' refers to the control of symptoms by the use of medications and non-pharmacological interventions. If the underlying cause is the cancer, it remains unchecked. This meaning is closest to the original Latin root 'pallium', a cloak. Oncologists use the term 'palliative' to refer to treatment which slows down or shrinks the cancer at one or more sites for as long as possible, with no expectation of cure. Symptoms are relieved for as long as the cancer remains in check. The latter meaning will pertain throughout this chapter.

Radiotherapy

Radiotherapy is the administration of various types of radiation, either from machines outside the body, or applied directly into or close by a cancer. It has a high chance of curing some localized cancers such as Hodgkin's lymphoma, laryngeal carcinoma, and cervical carcinoma.

Radiotherapy can also facilitate the symptomatic management of haemoptysis and cough due to endobronchial tumour, metastatic bone pain, and selected cases of spinal cord compression Patients with headaches and neurological deficits from intracerebral tumours or metastases may be considered for treatment. Control of rectal discharge or recurrent vaginal bleeding may be achieved for advanced inoperable pelvic cancers. Some doctors will treat pain associated with advanced head and neck tumours, dysphagia from advanced oesophageal cancer, and extensive soft tissue infiltration or ulceration, particularly from advanced, locally recurrent breast cancer.

A histological diagnosis of the cancer is almost always a prerequisite for treatment. If a diagnosis has not been made, an operation or other biopsy technique will be used. This principle may be waived if the patient has advanced disease, or abnormal non-invasive tests are consistent with the expected clinical pattern of metastatic disease and the risk of the biopsy is too great.

Efforts will frequently be made to identify how widespread the cancer is—a process known as staging. This may seem to expose the patient to a number of unnecessary tests but if the cancer is found to have spread to other important organs, such as liver or lung, lower doses of treatment may be used to reduce toxicity, or systemic hormone or chemotherapy may be considered. If the intention is merely to palliate the cancer at one site, staging is unnecessary. Even then, investigations may reveal other potential trouble spots such as impending fractures. These can then be treated before the patient develops more complex problems.

Patients who have very widespread disease and who are very ill will often not be considered for treatment. They find it difficult to be transported even short distances. Furthermore, they may not live long enough for the radiation to have a clinical effect.

When a decision is made to give radiotherapy, the treatment is carefully planned. Considerable care is needed to minimize radiation damage to normal tissues, especially in areas previously treated. Treatment is usually given by a number of doses (fractions) over a period of time, ranging from days to weeks. This reduces side-effects and, theoretically, increases the effect on the cancer. Some radiotherapists prescribe short courses, even single doses, when they are palliating symptoms in patient with advanced cancer who are relatively weak and cannot tolerate prolonged courses of treatment. Painful bone metastases are often treated this way. Long-term effects are unlikely to occur if the prognosis is short (Arnott 1987). Not all therapists agree with this approach, and it is important to be aware of the attitudes of individual radiotherapists.

In general, the side-effects of radiation treatment are now less frequent and less severe than in the past because of the advances made in the delivery of radiation, and the understanding of radiobiology. Many older patients will need reassurance because they will recall friends or relatives who suffered from treatment given many years ago. Acute effects include nausea and vomiting, particularly when the bowel is irradiated. Diarrhoea may also be a problem from abdominal or pelvic radiotherapy. Inflammation and dryness of the mouth can be especially troublesome during treatment of head and neck tumours, as can the burning retrosternal pain of oesophagitis when the mediastinum is treated. Some degree of alopecia, which is usually reversible, is invariable with cranial irradiation.

It is important to be aware of late effects which mimic the symptoms of advanced cancer and lead to patients being referred for terminal care. Fistula formation and cachexia from malabsorption after pelvic radio-therapy are examples. The pain of radiation-induced nerve damage may mimic malignant infiltration. The breathlessness and cough of post-radiation pneumonititis may be difficult to distinguish from the symptoms of primary lung cancer or lymphangitis carcinomatosis.

Hormone and chemotherapy

Hormone therapy is the use of hormones, such as oestrogens or progestagens, or drugs which block the production or effect of hormones, such as aminogluthemide and tamoxifen. The growth of some cancers will be affected by hormone manipulation. Chemotherapy refers to the use of drugs which can damage cancer cells directly.

The patients who present for chemotherapy represent a select group. Elderly patients, and patients with concomitant major illness, are usually not referred. The philosophy of the primary medical or surgical team which made the diagnosis will be a pre-selection factor. Many physicians and surgeons recall the toxicity of earlier treatments and will make an arbitrary decision not to refer. Many patients will accept such advice but a percentage will not, particularly the younger patients. A recent study by Slevin *et al.* (1988) revealed that patients referred for chemotherapy will accept a less than 1% chance of cure or relief of symptoms, despite potentially toxic treatment. Patients were prepared to accept a slimmer chance than the professionals who were caring for them.

When a patient first presents for consideration of hormone or chemotherapy, a diagnosis will usually have been made by means of a biopsy and examination of cancer tissue (histology). This prevents patients with non-malignant disorders from receiving potentially life-threatening treatment. To some extent, the histological diagnosis predicts the response of the cancer and this information plays an important part in the plan of the oncology team. Simple guidelines for the relative chances of cure and palliation for the more common forms of cancer is given in Table 8.1. This guideline does not imply that chemotherapy is the treatment of choice for these cancers in every situation.

To make decisions about treatment, oncologists use information about tumour response rates to various types of chemotherapy which is based on a large number of carefully performed studies. They also rely on anecdotal experience about patients who have survived despite the odds. Scenes of mutual celebration often occur when these patients attend clinics. These patients form a major counterpoise to the psychological effects of the deaths of so many others, and their example serves as an incentive for the doctors to encourage similar patients in the future. It is difficult to appreciate the importance of this experience when you first come into contact with an oncology service, particularly when you are primarily involved with the terminally ill patients.

The side-effects of treatment are another factor in the decision-making process. The majority of chemotherapy drugs will affect normal body tissues. Suppression of bone marrow function is common but usually reversible. Anaemia is slow to develop and can be easily treated with transfusions of red cells. A fall in the number of white cells and/or platelets may occur within days of treatment and is potentially far more serious.

Table 8.1 Guidelines of relative chances of cure and palliation for the more common forms of cancer

Definite chance of cure; good chance of palliation	Leukaemia (some types of childhood leukaemia) Lymphoma (Hodgkin's and some types of non-Hodgkin's lymphoma) Teratoma
Small chance of cure, good chance of palliation	Ovarian carcinoma Leukaemia (adult) Lymphoma (most types of non-Hodgkin's lymphoma)
Little/no chance of cure; good chance of palliation	Breast carcinoma Prostatic carcinoma Small-cell lung carcinoma
Little/no chance of cure; small chance of palliation	Colorectal and stomach carcinoma Pancreatic carcinoma Non-small-cell lung carcinoma Cervical carcinoma

Patients may die of overwhelming infections, or bleeding into the brain or bowel. Impairment of immunity may render patients more likely to infections such as shingles.

The commonest side-effects of chemotherapy are nausea and vomiting. These effects are now well controlled with the use of steroids and anti-emetic drugs when the chemotherapy is being administered. However, nausea may still be a problem 3–5 days following administration. If this the case patients whould be encouraged to continue their anti-emetics for the first week. Hair loss is also quite common and very distressing. Patients are also very distressed by the thought of coming for treatment, the time taken for treatment, and fear of needles (Coates *et al* 1983). Some patients will experience general effects such as lethargy and anorexia for several months after treatment. Individual agents may produce specific side-effects, such as peripheral neuritis caused by vincristine.

When there is a definite possibility of cure, doctors and patients will accept more side-effects and a greater risk of dying from the treatment. However, one of the major advances in oncology has been the recognition that, in a proportion of cancers, treatment toxicity can be reduced without jeopardizing response rates. This has resulted in shorter courses of treatment with fewer side-effects.

Another factor that is weighed up is the age of the patient. Older patients tolerate chemotherapy less well and are more likely to have other major illnesses. Younger patients may have a greater desire to pursue treatment at any cost, and the plight of these patients, particularly if they have young families, frequently mitigates a more aggressive response.

After considering the aforementioned factors, oncologists make one of the three decisions.

- No treatment. If a decision is made that no treatment is available or should be given, the patient will usually be discharged.
- No treatment but observe. This decision is usually made when patients have no symptoms and there is a poor chance of the disease responding to known treatments. Patients may be offered the option of review in the out-patient clinic until symptoms develop.
- Proceed with treatment. This decision may include a distinction between an attempt to cure or to palliate the cancer.

When a decision is made for treatment, further tests are usually done to stage the cancer and measure the size of cancer deposits. The results serve as a baseline to assess if treatment is effective, and may influence the type of treatment to be used. Many investigations, such as blood tests, are carried out routinely, often according to a pre-planned protocol. In a situation where there is a distinct probability of cure, investigations may involve more discomfort and greater risk to patients. Additional investigations may be ordered depending on patient symptoms or unexpected findings from routine tests.

The number and nature of investigations may be reduced if the patient is too unwell or if a life-threatening delay in treatment might result. Where treatment is palliative with a relatively small chance of response, tests will often be kept to a minimum. Oncology units which research and compare various treatment protocols will rarely modify a rigid programme of investigations. This policy may seem callous and inflexible but it has resulted in the considerable improvements in the quality of life afforded to patients receiving palliative treatment.

Most units will have standard treatments depending on the diagnosis and stage of the disease. Some chemotherapeutic agents are used continuously. The majority of cytotoxic drugs are given as a course of injections and/or tablets which are repeated at regular intervals.

Once a patient has been commenced on treatment, they are usually subject to ongoing reviews. If the cancer is physically apparent, the tumour will be measured before each course of treatment is due. After two or three courses of treatment, tests which demonstrate the size of the cancer will be repeated—it often takes several weeks before a response is apparent. If the cancer is responding, therapy will be continued for a set number of treatments or until the cancer is not detectable.

If the cancer progresses through treatment, another aggressive protocol will be used if there is a chance of cure. If this is not feasible or appropriate, therapy will often de-escalate to less intensive palliative treatment. Severe side-effects may lead to a change in, or cessation of treatment, even when the disease is responding.

Response to treatment is not always reviewed. In some instances, such as metastatic bone disease, objective response will lag several weeks behind subjective improvement. It may not be possible to quantitate response in some patients. On other occasions, doctors will continue with treatment without attempting to assess disease because they do not want to know if the cancer is progressing; they want to maintain the patient's hope in the treatment.

The majority of oncology units will provide supportive medical care throughout treatment. Patients and families are educated about symptoms which herald low platelet or white cell count. Regular blood tests will be performed between courses. However, the oncology team may not be as aware of distressing symptoms, such as nausea and vomiting, which are not life-threatening. Patients will frequently underestimate the severity of symptoms which occur between courses.

Increasing attention is being paid to the emotional support of patients and their families. Nursing staff and other patients play an important role in this regard. Some units employ oncology nurse specialists or social workers. Support groups—informal meetings of patients, families, and staff—for site-specific cancers such as breast, brain, and head and neck cancers are now quite common. Formal psychological support services may also be available.

Some cancer centres have built or developed cancer information offices for the lay public nearby the treatment centre (Young 1993; Wood 1994). Such enterprises have proved extremely popular and are developing their own complimentary aspects of care. Information booklets such as those produced by BACUP (London) on the different cancers, aspects of physical and psychological care, as well as the emotional affects of the family throughout the illness are now widely distributed.

Patients receiving chemotherapy will frequently be given more information about their disease and the treatment than is usually the case in other diseases or treatments. Doctors assume that patients require to know their diagnosis and treatment prospects in order to cooperate fully with potentially toxic therapy. But it is interesting to note how many patients who are not told their diagnosis will submit to such treatment (Gould and Toghill 1981). Doctors present information at interviews and ward rounds. Oncology nurse specialists will supplement this knowledge.

McGrath and Kearsley (1995) propose an interesting concept of 'best supportive care' clinics being an alternative for patients receiving palliative chemotherapy when any therapeutic result from further chemotherapy is unlikely to be achieved. Unfortunately further palliative chemotherapy can sometimes be used as an excuse for tackling difficult end-of-life discussions.

Working with oncology services

Oncologists and radiotherapists will have many patients who are likely to die despite treatment, and the palliative care team is often asked to be involved with these patients. The following guidelines are offered to facilitate relations between oncology services and the hospital-based palliative care team.

1. Determine if you can work alongside 'active' treatment. Some teams have tried to help patients to accept impending death rather than pressing on with further 'futile' courses of treatment. Many patients have been angered by this approach and transferred their anger to the primary team for asking the palliative care team to be involved. This has made the oncology team reluctant to refer other patients. Some patients are referred because of deterioration during treatment, before a response is apparent. The doctors will often want to continue therapy, and this decision to refer will cause them considerable stress (Degner and Beaton 1987). Such stress will be compounded if the team member seeks to prevent further treatment being given. If the needs of the patient have not been properly ascertained, it may be more prudent to avoid raising such issues. If these situations become too difficult, it may be easier to limit the team's role to those patients who are definitely not having further treatment.

2. Recognize skills that oncologists have in terminal care. It is important to avoid any sense of rivalry that may develop when oncology services incorporate basic concepts of symptom relief and supportive care into their clinical practice.

3. Maintain an open approach with patients who are seeking further active treatment or who are being treated. It is important to listen to

what the patient wants, and facilitate this as far as is possible. This involves supporting the patient's desire for an oncology opinion if the primary team have dismissed this option. When listening to patients who are receiving treatment, remember that 'I do not like chemo-therapy' does not equate with 'I do not want chemotherapy'. Patients often like to share their frustrations about having no options except therapy, but be careful about how you interpret these frustrations.

4. Report information about the patient's quality of life. Maintaining regular contact with out-patients makes one more aware of the incidence and severity of side-effects. This information should be reported either directly to the oncologist or in the medical notes. This will often facilitate better control of symptoms during treatment. The patient may need encouragement to seek readmission if there are life-threatening side-effects.

5. Identify who makes decisions about patient treatment. Decisions relating to the initiation or discontinuation of treatment usually rest with the consultant or senior registrar. One will need to approach them if the patient genuinely wishes to stop therapy. However, decisions about minor modifications in analgesics and other medications for symptom control may be made by the junior doctors.

6. Identify where decisions are made. Decisions about in-patients will often be made or ratified during formal ward rounds. These rounds can be daunting unless you accompany them routinely. Informal ward rounds are a less intimidating forum, particularly for issues pertaining to symptom control. Combined clinics and meetings bring together several disciplines to discuss problem cases. Where possible, these meetings should be attended; they provide an ideal opportunity to raise points about terminal care, and other teams will become familiar with your work.

7. Be aware of the doctors' individual preferences about treatments. Time should be spent with the nearest oncology unit, during orientation to the palliative care team, becoming aware of the referral pattern of the physicians and surgeons who use these services. When working closely with a unit, do not presume on one's own familiarity with the different approaches that doctors have to treatment. A relationship with a patient may be jeopardized if an alternative treatment programme is decided upon.

8. Facilitate the transfer of distressing information. Hinton (1979) observed on one radiotherapy unit that there was a relative lack of frank discussion about dying. This did not appear to relate to pressures

on time. He postulated that it was due to the emotional investment required when treating patients. This commitment made it difficult for carers to adjust to treatment failure. The palliative care team can be in a better position to pick up on issues relating to disease progression.

It is often thought that patients receiving anti-cancer therapy cannot come to terms with their diagnosis because they are constantly focusing on the hopeful outcome of treatment. A small minority of patients deny their illness, but most will recognize when their cancer is progressing through treatment. They are very aware of lumps increasing in size, deterioration in their general health and specific symptoms, and subtle changes in the way the primary team relates to them.

Although patients are more likely to know their diagnosis and what treatment entails, information about the likelihood and consequences of treatment failure is less forthcoming. This applies particularly when curative treatment is considered, but often applies to palliative therapy. Many patients will want confirmation about the progress of their illness, and it can be helpful to get the primary team to review test results with them. It is gratifying how readily doctors will include this information when they realize that the patient wants it (Reynolds *et al.* 1981). Confirmation that the cancer is progressing will frequently precipitate opportunities to tackle fears and unresolved burdens. The patient will not necessarily want to abandon treatment.

The introduction of the idea of attending a local day hospice for some patients who have been attending the clinic for several years can be useful. It gives them a different angle on which to look at their cancer especially if the day hospice is well supported by medical staff and can be available for symptom control advice. It may also help the oncologist to step back from giving still further chemotherapy. For some patients it is not so much a fear of stopping chemotherapy as a fear that no one will be interested in them any more if they decide to stop treatment.

Epilogue

These guidelines should give some insight into the advantages that result from an atmosphere of mutual cooperation. Managing the distress and the symptoms of advancing cancer, and being prepared to work alongside the primary team, will greatly reassure patients. Families and the professional carers will also appreciate the extra dimension of supportive care that can be offered. This will allow you to become part of a truly integrated service; a service offering a balanced approach to patients and families who are struggling to come to terms with the devastating impact of advanced cancer.

Death must simply become the discreet but dignified exit of a peaceful person from a helpful society, without pain or suffering, and ultimately without fear. (Philippe Airies, *The Hour of Our Death*, 1997)

References

Abraham, J.L., Callahan, J., Rossetti, K., and Pierre, L. (1996) The impact of a hospice consultation team on the care of veterans with advanced cancer. *Journal of Pain and Symptom Management*, **12**(1), 23–31.

Addington-Hall, J.M., MacDonald, L.D., Anderson, H.R. and Freeling, P. (1991) Dying from cancer: the views of bereaved family and friends about the experiences of terminally ill patients *Palliative Medicine*, **5**, 207–14.

Ahmedzai, S. (1982) Dying in hospital: the residents' viewpoint. *British Medical Journal*, **285**, 712.

Arnott, S. (1987) The role of radiotherapy in treatment of metastatic cancer. In:*Management of metastases. Ballière's clinical oncology—international practice and research*, Vol. 1 (ed. M.L. Slevin), pp. 537–50. Ballière Tindall, London.

Ajemain, I. (1993) The interdisciplinary team. In *The Oxford textbook of palliative medicine*. (ed. D. Doyle, G. Hanks, and N. Macdonald). Oxford University Press, Oxford.

Axelsson, B. and Borup Christensen, S. (1996) Place of death correlated to sociodemographic factors: a study of 203 patients dying of cancer in a rural Swedish county in 1990. *Palliative Medicine*, **10**, 329–35.

Bales, R.F. (1950) *Interaction process analysis*. Addison Wesley, Reading, Mass.

Bascom, P.B. (1997) A hospital-based comfort care team: consultation for seriously ill and dying patients. *American Journal of Hospice and Palliative Care*, **14**(2), 57—61.

Bates, T.D. (1985) *St Thomas Hospital Terminal Care Support Team: eighth annual report*. Available from the Secretary, Palliative Care Team, St Thomas' Hospital, London SE1 7EH.

Bates, T.D., Hoy, A.M., Clarke, D.G., and Laird, P.P. (1981) The St Thomas Hospital Terminal Care Support Team—a new concept of hospice care. *Lancet*, i, 1201–3.

Beauchamp, T.L. and Childrees, J.F. (1983) *Principles of biomedical ethics*, 2nd edn. Oxford University Press, New York.

Beckhard, R. (1974) Organizational implications of team building. In *Making healthcare teams work*, pp 69–98 (ed. H. Wise, R. Beckhard, I. Rubin and A.L. Kyte). Ballinger, Cambridge, MA.

Bennett, M. and Corcoran, G. (1994) The impact on community palliative care services of a hospital palliative care team. *Palliative Medicine*, **8**, 237–44.

Billings, J.A. (1985) *Outpatient management of advanced cancer*. Lippincott, Philadelphia, PA.

Boas, R.A. (1983) The sympathetic nervous system and pain relief. In *Relief of Intractable Pain* (ed. M. Swerdlow). pp. 215–37. Elsevier, Amsterdam.

Bolam v. Friern Hospital Management Committee. 1 W.L.R. 582.

Bowling, A. (1983) The hospitalisation of death: should more people die at home? *Journal of Medical Ethics*, 9, 158–61.

Bowling, A. and Cartwright, A. (1982) *Life after death: a study of the elderly widowed.* Routledge and Kegan Paul, London.

Bragg, M. (1996) *Reinventing influence: How to get things done in a world without authority* Pitman, London.

Brazil, K. and Thomas, D. (1995) The role of volunteers in a hospital-based palliative care service. *Journal of Palliative Care*, 11(3), 40–2.

Brescia, F.J., Adler, D., Gray, G. *et al.* (1990) Hospitalized advanced cancer patients: a profile. *Journal of Pain and Symptom Management*, 5, 221–7.

Bristow, A. and Foster, J.M.G. (1988) Lumbar sympathectomy in the management of rectal tenesmoid pain. *Annals of the Royal College of Surgeons of England*, 70, 38–9.

Bruera, E. (1993) Research in symptoms other than pain. In *Oxford textbook of palliative medicine* (ed. D, Doyle, G. Hanks and N. MacDonald), p 87. Oxford University Press, Oxford.

Bruera, E., Brenneis, C., Michaud, M., and MacDonald, N. (1989) Influence of the Pain and Symptom Control Team (PSCT) on the patterns of treatment of pain and other symptoms in a cancer center. *Journal of Pain and Symptom Management*, 4(3),112–16.

Bruera, E., Kuehn, N., Miller, M.J., Selmser, P., and Macmillan K. (1991) The Edmonton Symptom Assessment System (ESAS). A simple method for the assessment of palliative care patients *Journal of Palliative Care*, 7(2), 6–9.

Buckman, R. (1984) Breaking bad news: why is it still so difficult? *British Medical Journal*, 288, 1597–9.

Calman, K., and Hine, D. (1995) *A policy framework for commissioning cancer services*. Department of Health, London, UK.

Cartwright, A., Hockey, L., and Anderson, J.L. (1973) *Life before death*. Routledge and Kegan Paul, London.

Cartwright, A. (1991) Balance of care for the dying between hospitals and the community: perceptions of general practitioners, hospital consultants, community nurses and relatives. *British Journal of General Practice*, 41, 271–4.

Charlton, J.E. (1986) Current views on the use of nerve blocking in the relief of chronic pain. In: *The therapy of pain* (2nd ed) pp. 133–64.

Chochinov, H., Wilson, K.G., Enns, M., Mowchun, N., Lander, S., Levitt, M., and Clinch, J.J. (1995) Desire for death in the terminally ill. *American Journal of Psychiatry*, 152, 1185–91.

Coates, A., Abraham, S., Kaye, S.B. *et al.* (1983) On the receiving end—patient perception of the side-effects of cancer chemotherapy. *European Journal of Cancer and Clinical Oncology*, 19, 203–8.

Colquhoun, M., and Dougan, H. (1997) Ensuring that the specialist nurse is special. *Palliative Medicine*, 11, 381–7.

Cook, M. (1988) A guide to staff selection techniques for the NHS in Wales: uses and abuses of psychometric testing. Cardiff, Welsh Health Service.

Cousins, M.J., Cherry, D.A., and Gourlay, G.K. Acute and chronic pain: use of spinal opiods. In *Neural Blockade in Clinical Anaesthesia and Management of Pain,* 2nd edn (ed. M.J. Cousins and P.O. Bridenbaugh), pp 955–1029. Lippincott, Philadelphia.

Crowther, T. (1993) Euthanasia. In *The future for palliative care: issues of policy and practice* (ed. D. Clark). Open University Press, Buckingham.

Degner, L. and Beaton, J.I. (1987) *Life–death decisions in health care.* Hemisphere, Washington, DC.

Dunlop, R. and Hockley, J. (1991) Efficiency versus compassion in the National Health Service *Palliative Medicine,* 5(1), 1–3.

Dunlop, R., Hockley, J., and Davies, R.J. (1989) Preferred versus actual place of death—a hospital terminal care support team experience. *Palliative Medicine,* 3, 197–201.

Dunphy, K., Finley, I., Rathbone, G., Gilbert, J., and Hicks, F. (1995) Rehydration in palliative and terminal care: if not—why not? *Palliative Medicine,* 9, 221–8.

Ellershaw, J., Peat, S.J., and Boys, L.C. (1995) Assessing the effectiveness of a hospital palliative care team *Palliative Medicine,* 9, 145–52.

Fainsinger, R.L. (1997) How often can we justify parenteral nutrition in terminally ill cancer patients ? *Journal of Palliative Care,* 13(1), 48–51.

Field, D., and James, N. (1993) Where and how people die. In: *The future of palliative care: issues of policy and practice* (ed: Clark, D.) Open University Press, Buckingham.

Filshie, J. (1990) Acupuncture and malignant pain problems. *Acupuncture in Medicine,* 8, 38–9.

Fineman, S.P. Long-term post-thoracotomy cancer pain management with interpleural bupivacaine. *Anaesthesia and Analgesia,* 68, 694–7.

Finley, I.G. and Jones, R.V.H. (1995) Outreach palliative care services: definitions in palliative care. *British Medical Journal,* 311, 754.

Firth, S. (1993) Cultural issues in terminal care. In *The future for palliative care—issues of policy and practice* (ed. D. Clark). Open University Press, Buckingham.

Foster, J.M.G. (1990) The pain clinic. In *Terminal Care Support Teams: the hospital/hospice interface* (ed. R.J. Dunlop and J.M. Hockley), pp. 75–82. Oxford University Press, Oxford.

Gillon, R. (1994) Medical ethics: four principles plus attention to scope. *British Medical Journal,* 309, 184–8.

Greenhill, V.M. (1996) The value of research in assessing the need for a palliative care team in the hospital setting. *Journal of Cancer Care,* 5, 169–72.

Greer, D.S., Mor, V., Morris, J.N., Sherwood, S., Kidder, D., and Birnbaum, H.

(1986) An alternative in terminal care: results of the National Hospice Study. *Journal of Chronic Diseases*, **39**, 9–26.

Goldman, A. and Baum, D. (1994) Provision of care In *Care of the dying child* (ed. A. Goldman). Oxford University Press, Oxford.

Gould, H. and Toghill, P.J. (1981) How should we talk about acute leukaemia to adult patients and their families? *British Medical Journal*, **282**, 210–12.

Hector, W. (1974) Nursing. In *The Royal Hospital of St Bartholomew* (ed. V.C. Medvei and J.L. Thornton), p. 460. Cavell, London.

Herd, E.B. (1990) Terminal care in a semi-rural area. *British Journal of General Practice*, **40**, 248–251.

Herth, K. (1990) Fostering hope in terminally-ill people. *Journal of Advanced Nursing*, **15**, 1250–9.

Herxheimer, A., Begent, R., MacLean, D., Phillips, L., Southcott, B. and Walton, I. (1985) Short life of a terminal care support team: experience at Charing Cross Hospital. *British Medical Journal*, **290**, 1877–9.

Higginson, I.J., Wade, A.M., and McCarthy, M. (1992) Effectiveness of two palliative support teams. *Journal of Public Health Medicine*, **14**(1), 50–6.

Hilton, A. (1990) This house believes that there is a role for euthanasia in cancer care. *Cancer nursing—the balance. Proceedings of the 6th international conference on cancer nursing* (ed. A.P. Pritchard). Scutari Press, London.

Hinton, J. (1963) The physical and mental distress of the dying. *Quarterly Journal of Medicine*, **32**, 1–21.

Hinton, J. (1979) Comparison of places and policies for terminal care. *Lancet*, i, 29–32.

Hockley, J. (1989) Caring for the dying in acute hospitals. *Nursing Times*, **85**, 47–50.

Hockley, J. (1993) The concept of hope and the will to live. *Palliative Medicine*, **7**, 181–6.

Hockley, J. (1996) The development of a palliative care team at the Western General Hospital, Edinburgh. *Supportive Care in Cancer*, **4**, 77–81.

Hockley, J., Dunlop, R., and Davies, R.J. (1998) Survey of distressing symptoms in dying patients and their families in hospital and the response to a symptom control team. *British Medical Journal*, **296**, 1715–17.

Hoskins, P. and Hanks, G. (1988) Management of symptoms in advanced cancer: experience in a hospital-based continuing care unit. *Journal of the Royal Society of Medicine*, **81**, 341–4.

House of Commons (1992) *Notices of Motions*, 20 January, No. 43, 1571.

Houtes, P.S., Yasko, J.M., Harvey, H.A., Kahn, S.B., Hartz, A.J., Hermann, J.F., *et al.* (1988) Unmet needs of persons with cancer in Pennsylvania during the period of terminal care. *Cancer*, **62**, 627–34.

Hoy, A.M., Saunders, B.M., and Kearney, M. (1984) Breaking bad news. *British Medical Journal*, **288**, 1833.

Hyett, K. (1984) Effective panel interviewing. *Nursing Times,* **80,** 1 February, 47–8.

Jarvis, H., Burge, F.I., and Scott C.A. (1996) Evaluating a palliative care program: methodology and limitations. *Journal of Palliative Care,* 12(2), 23–33.

Jeffrey, D. (1993) *There is nothing more I can do—an introduction to the ethics of palliatve care.* Lisa Sainsbury Foundation, Patten Press, Cornwall.

Johnson, D.W. and Johnson, F.P. (1975) *Joining together: Group theory and group skills.* New Jersey, Prentice-Hall, Inc.

Kaplan, M.P. and O'Connor, P. (1989) Hospice care for minorities: an analysis of a hospital-based inner city palliative care service *American Journal of Hospice Care,* **6,** 13–21.

Kelly, W.D. and Friesen, S.R. (1950) Do cancer patients want to be told? *Surgery,* **27,** 322–26: cited by R.Weir in *Moral Problems in Medecine,* 2nd edn (ed. S. Gorovitz, R. Macklin, A.L. Jameton, J.M. O'Connor and ? Sherwin), p. 204. Prentice-Hall, Englewood Cliffs, NJ.

Knight, M. and Field, D. (1981) A silent conspiracy: coping with dying cancer patients on an acute surgical ward. *Journal of Advanced Nursing,* **6,** 221–9.

Kristjanson, L.J. (1986) Indicators of quality of palliative care from a family perspective. *Journal of Palliative Care,* **1,** 8–17.

LaGrand, L.E. (1980) Reducing burnout in the hospice and the death education movement. *Death Education,* **4,** 61–75.

Lassauniere, J. (1994) A mobile palliative care team. *European Journal of Palliative Care,* 1(3), 130–1.

Latimer, E. (1991) Caring for seriously ill and dying patients: philosophy and ethics. *Canadian Medical Association Journal,* **144** (7), 859–64.

Lewin, K., Lippitt, R., and White, R.K. (1939) Patterns of aggressive behaviour in experimentally created social climates. *Journal of Social Psychology* **10,** 271–299. Cited by Johnson, D.W. and Johnson, F.P. (1975) *Joining together: Group theory and group skills.* New Jersey, Prentice-Hall, Inc.

Lipton, S. (1979) Current views on the therapy of chronic pain. Percutaneous cervical cordotomy and the injection of the pituitary with alcohol. *Anaesthesia,* **33,** 953–7.

Lunt, B. and Hillier, R. (1981) Terminal care: present services and future priorities. *British Medical Journal,* **283,** 595–8.

MacAdam, D.B. and Smith, M. (1987) An initial assessment of suffering in terminal illness. *Palliative Medicine,* **1,** 37–47.

McCorkle, R. and Young, K. (1978) Development of a symptom distress scale. *Cancer Nursing* **1,** 373–8.

McCue, J.D. (1982) The effects of stress on physicians and their medical practice. *New England Journal of Medicine,* **306,** 458–63.

McGrath, P. and Kearsley, J.H. (1995) Is there a better way? Bioethical reflections on palliative cytotoxic drug use (editorial). *Palliative Medicine,* **9,** 269–71.

Maguire, P. (1985) Barriers to psycholgocial care of the dying. *British Medical Journal*, 291, 1711–13.

McQuay, H. and Moore, A. (1994) Need for rigorous assessment of palliative care. *British Medical Journal*, **309**, 1315–16.

McQuillan, R., Finley, I., Branch, C., Roberts, D., and Spencer, M. (1996) Improving analgesic prescribing in a general teaching hospital *Journal of Pain and Symptom Management*, 11(3), 172–5.

McWhinney, I.R., Bass, M.J., Donner, A. (1994) Evaluation of palliative care services problems and pitfalls. *British Medical Journal*, **309**, 1340–42.

Meyerson, B.A. (1990) Electrical stimulation of spinal cord and brain. In *The management of pain*, 2nd edn (ed. J.J Bonica), pp. 1862–7. Lea and Febiger, Philadelphia, PA.

Moore, N. (1918) *The history of St Bartholomews Hospital*. Pearson, London.

Morris, W.A. (1981) Care of the terminally ill in a district general hospital. *British Medical Journal*, **282**, 287–8.

Mount, B.M., Jones, A. and Patterson, A. (1974) Death and dying: attitudes in a teaching hospital. *Urology*, 4, 741–7.

Mount, B.M. (1980) Personal selection, applying the McMurray principles to palliative care. In *The RVH.manual on palliative/hospice care* (ed. I. Ajemian and B.M. Mount), pp 21–6. Arno Press, New York.

NAHA (1987) *Care of the dying—a guide for health authorities*. National Association of Health Authorities, 4 Edgbaston Park Road, Birmingham B13 2RS.

Nash, T.P. (1984) Breaking bad news. *British Medical Journal*, **288**, 1996.

NCHSPCS (1993) *Key Ethical Issues in Palliative Care: Evidence to House of Lords Select Committee on Medical Ethics*. Occasional Paper 3. National Council for Hospice and Specialist Palliative Care Services, 59 Bryanston Street, London W1A 2AZ.

Normand, C. (1996) Economics and evaluation of palliative care (editorial). *Palliative Medicine*, 10(1), 3–4.

NWTHRA (1987). *Regional strategy—towards a strategy for dying and bereaved people*. North West Thames Regional Health Authority, 40 Eastbourne Terrace, London, W2 3QR.

Office of Population Censuses and Surveys (1989) *Mortality statistics for 1987. England and Wales*. HMSO, London.

Oken, D. (1961) What to tell cancer patients. *Journal of American Medical Association*, 175, 1120–8.

O'Neil, W.M., O'Connor, P. and Latimer, E.J. (1992) Hospital palliative care services: three models in three countries. *Journal of Pain and Symptom Management*, 7(7), 406–13.

Ostrowski, M.J. (1979) Pain control in advanced malignant disease using transcutaneous nerve stimulation. *British Journal of Clinical Practice*, 33, 157–62.

Oxenham, D. and Boyd, D. (1997) Voluntary euthanasia in terminal illness. In *New themes in palliative care* (ed. D. Clark, J. Hockley and S. Amhedzai). Open University Press, Buckingham.

Parkes, C.M. (1985) Terminal care: home, hospital or hospice? *Lancet*, i, 155–7.

Plancarte, R., Amescua, C., Patt, R.B. and Aldrete, J.A. (1990a) Superior hypogastric plexus block for pelvic cancer pain *Anesthesiology*, 73, 236–9.

Plancarte, R., Amescua, C., Patt, R.B. and Aldrete, J.A. (1990b) Presacral blockade of the ganglion of Walther (ganglion impar) *Anesthesiology*, 73, A751.

Plumbley, P. (1991) *Recruitment and selection*, 5th edn. Billing and Sons, Worcester, MA.

Raftery, J.P., Addington-Hall, J.M., MacDonald, L.D. *et al.* (1996) A randomized controlled trial of the effectiveness of a district co-ordinating service for terminally ill cancer patients *Palliative Medicine*, 10(2), 151–61.

Rainey, L.C., Crane, L.A., Breslow, D.M. and Ganz, P.A. (1980) Cancer patients' attitudes toward hospice services *Ca: A Cancer Journal for Clinicians*, 34, 191–201.

RCPCH. (1997) *A guide to the development of children palliative care services*. A report of joint working party of the Association for Children with Life Threatening and Terminal Condition and their Family. ACT., 65 St Michaels Hill, Bristol BS2 8DZ.

Reynolds, P.M., Sanson-Fisher, R.W., Desmond Pool, A., Harber J., and Byrne, M.J. (1981) Cancer and communication: information giving on an oncology clinic. *British Medical Journal*, 282, 1449–51.

Robbins, M. (1997) Assessing needs and effectiveness: is palliative care a special case? In *New themes in palliative care* (ed. D. Clark, J. Hockley, and S. Ahmedzai). Open University Press: Buckingham.

Roisin, D., Laval, G., and Lelut, B. (1994) Interdisciplinary activity in a mobile palliative care team. *European Journal of Palliative Care*, 1(3), 132–5.

Saltzburg, D. and Foley, K.M. (1989) Management of pain in pancreatic cancer. *Surgical Clinics of North America*, 69, 629–49.

Saunders, C. (1980) Caring to the end. *Nursing Mirror*. Sept 4. p. 52.

Saunders, C. (1986) Current views on pain relief and terminal care. In *The therapy of pain*, 2nd edn (ed. M. Swerdlow), pp. 239–59. MTP Press, Lancaster.

Saunders, C. (1988) The evolution of the hospice. In: *The history of the management of pain: from early principles to present practice* (ed R.D. Mann). Partheman Publishing Group, Carnforth.

Saunders, C. (1993) History and challenge In *The management of terminal malignant disease* (ed. C. Saunders and N. Sykes), p. 6. Edward Arnold, London.

Senge, P. (1990) *The fifth discipline: The art and practice of the learning organisation*. Currency Doubleday, New York.

Sidaway v. Bethlem Board of Governors (1985). 2 W.L.R. 480 (HL).

Simpson, K.H. (1991) The use of research to facilitate the creation of a hospital palliative care team. *Palliative Medicine,* 5, 122–9.

Slevin, M.L., Plant, H., Lynch, D., Drinkwater, J., and Gregory W.M. (1988) Who should measure quality of life, the doctor or the patient? *British Journal of Cancer,* 57, 109–12.

Smith, N. (1990) The impact of terminal illness on the family. *Palliative Medicine* 4(2), 127–35.

Spiegel, D. (1985) The use of hypnosis in controlling cancer pain. *Cancer Journal for Clinicans,* 4, 221–31.

St Christopher's Hospice Information Service/Directory. (1997) Obtained from: St Christopher's Hospice, Sydenham, London SE26 6DZ.

Stokes, J., Wyer, S., and Crossley, D. (1997) The challenge of evaluating a child bereavement programme. *Palliative Medicine,* 11(3), 179–90.

Thelen, H.A. (1965) *Dynamics of groups at work* (7th impression) Chicago: University of Chicago Press, pp 197–332.

Tolstoy, L. (1960) *The Death of Ivan Ilyich* (English translation by Rosemary Edmonds). Penguin, Harmondsworth.

Townsend, J., Frank, A.O., Ferment, D., Dyer, S., Karran, O., Walgrove, A., and Piper, M. (1990) Terminal cancer care and patients' preference for place of death: a prospective study. *British Medical Journal,* 301, 415–17.

van der Maas, P.J., van Delden, J.M., Pijnenborg, L., and Looman, C.W.N. Euthanasia and other medical decisions concerning the end of life. *Lancet,* 338, 669–74.

Vachon, M.L.S. (1978) Moviation and stress experienced by staff working with the terminally ill. *Death Education,* 2, 113–22.

Vachon, M.L.S. (1986) Battle fatigue in hospice/palliative care. In *1986 International symposium on pain control* (ed D. Doyle), pp. 69–76. International congress and symposium series, Royal Society of Medicine, London.

Vachon, M.L.S. (1987) *Occupational stress in the care of the critically ill, the dying and the bereaved.* Hemisphere, Washington.

Wales, J., Kane, R., Robbins, S., Bernstein, L., and Krasnow, R. (1983) UCLA Hospice evaluation study. *Medical Care,* 21(7), 734–44.

Weissman, D. and Griffie, J. (1994) The Palliative Care Consultation Service of the Medical College of Wisconsin. *Journal of Pain and Symptom Management,* 9(7), 474—9.

Whitfield, S.A. (1979) A descriptive study of student nurses' ward experience with dying patients and their attitudes towards them. Unpublished thesis, Manchester University.

WHO. (1990) *Cancer pain relief and palliative care.* Technical Report Series 804, World Health Organization, Geneva.

Wilkes, E. (1984) Dying now. *Lancet,* i, 950–2.

Wilkes, L., White, K., and Tolley, T. (1993) Euthanasia: a comparison of the lived experience of Chinese and Australian palliative care nurses. *Journal of Advanced Nursing*, 18, 95–102.

Wood, J. (1994) Support and information for cancer patients in the UK. *Radiography Today*, August, 60(687), 16–18.

Wright, A., Cousins, J., and Upward, J. (1988) *Matters of death and life. A study of bereavement support in NHS hospitals in England.* King Edward's Hospital Fund for London, London.

Young, J. (1993) New cancer support centre opens at Mount Vernon. *British Psycho-Oncology Group Newsletter*, September.

Yukl, G. and Falbe, CM. (1990) Influence tactics and objectives in upward, downward, and lateral influence attempts. *Journal of Applied Psychology*, 75, 132–40.

Appendix 1

Recommended reading

Billings, J.A. (1985) *Outpatient management of advanced cancer.* Lippincott, Philadelphia, PA.

Clark, D., Hockley, J. and Ahmedzai, S. (1997) *New themes in palliative care.* Open University Press, Buckingham.

Copperman, H, (1983) *Dying at home.* Wiley, Chichester.

Doyle, D., Hanks, G. and MacDonald, N. (1998) *Oxford textbook of palliative medicine,* 2nd edn. Oxford University Press, Oxford.

Saunders, C. and Sykes, N. (1993) *The managment of terminal malignant disease,* 3rd edn. Edward Arnold, London.

Stedeford, A. (1984) *Facing death.* Heinemann, London.

Twycross, R.G. (1997) *Symptom managment in advanced cancer,* 2nd edn. Radcliffe Medical, Oxford.

Vachon, M.L.S. (1987) *Occupational stress in the care of the critically ill, the care of the dying, and the bereaved.* Hemisphere, Washington.

Appendix 2

Sample Palliative Care Team Patient Information Form
WESTERN GENERAL HOSPITAL NHS TRUST, Edinburgh

Name	D.O.B.
Address	Marital Status S M Sep D W
	Ward / tel.
Tel.	Consultant
N.O.K. / Main Carer	G.P.
Address	Address
Tel.	Tel.
District Nurse	Social Worker
Tel.	Social Services
Home Care/Nurse specialists	

Referral information

Date of Referral	Date seen

Source of Referral:

Oncology	Medical Oncology	Radiotherapy	Haematology	
Medicine	General	Respiratory	Rheumatology	Infectious Diseases
Surgery	General	Urology		
Neuroscience	surgery	neurology		
RVH				

Reason for Referral:

Pain	symptom control	psychological support : patient / family
Discharge advice	staff support	bereavement support

Outcome

Discharge Date	Date of Death

Discharge to:	Hospice	Other hospital
	Home	Carer's home
	Nursing home	Other

. . . . /contd

Diagnosis

Histology

History   **X-rays/Scans**

Bloods

Hb   Urea   Creatinine
Albumen   Alk phos   Calcium   Others:

Medications

DRUG	On referral	DATE						

. . . . /contd

First Assessment

Insight into disease:

1. Accepts diagnosis + terminal condition (actual or potential)
2. Accepts diagnosis + aware of secondary spread but doesn't talk about dying
3. Accepts diagnosis + unaware of prognosis (death/disability)
4. Unsure about diagnosis
5. Expecting full recovery/significant denial
6. Not assessed (reason)

Main Problems:

1st Assessment	Score	2nd assessment	Score
1.		1.	
2.		2.	
3.		3.	

Patient /family reaction to diagnosis/prognosis

Genogram

Religion/spirituality

. . . . /contd

PAIN CHART

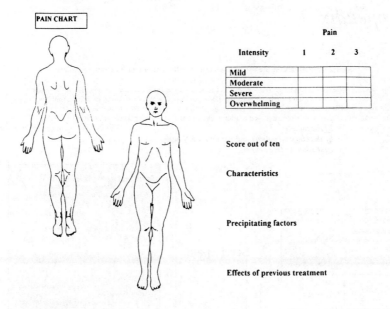

Pain

Intensity	1	2	3
Mild			
Moderate			
Severe			
Overwhelming			

Score out of ten

Characteristics

Precipitating factors

Effects of previous treatment

Current symptoms

	Absent	Mild	Moderate	Severe	Comments
Pain					
Anorexia					
Weight loss					
Indigestion					
Nausea/vomiting					
Constipation					
Diarrhoea					
Ascites					
Dyspnoea					
Weakness					
Drowsiness					
Insomnia					
Jaundice					
Oedema					
Cough					
Urinary symptoms					
OTHER SYMPTOMS					

Appendix 3

Sample guidelines on the use of analgesics for the patient with advanced cancer

The following information details the general principles and guidelines useful in the choice of analgesics for pain in patients with advanced cancer. It is essential that before any analgesics are chosen a detailed assessment of the patient's pain is performed. This must include details on: the exact site of the pain, the possible cause of the pain, the type of pain, and its severity. The World Health Organisation recommends that to achieve optimum pain relief analgesia must be given as follows:

- *by the mouth*
- *by the clock (regularly and not on a PRN basis)*
- *by the ladder (see below)*

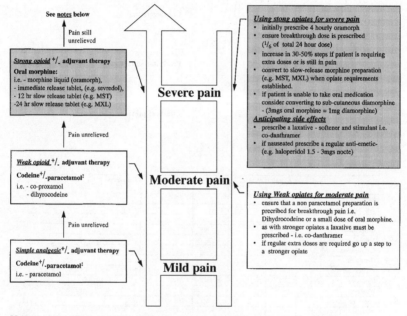

See **notes** below

Pain still
unrelieved

Strong opioid +/- adjuvant therapy

Oral morphine:
i.e. - morphine liquid (oramorph),
- immediate release tablet, (e.g. sevredol),
- 12 hr slow release tablet (e.g. MST)
- 24 hr slow release tablet (e.g. MXL)

Pain unrelieved

Weak opioid +/- adjuvant therapy

Codeine +/- paracetamol:
i.e. - co-proxamol
- dihyrocodeine

Pain unrelieved

Simple analgesic +/- adjuvant therapy

Codeine +/- paracetamol:
i.e. - paracetamol

Severe pain

Moderate pain

Mild pain

Using strong opiates for severe pain
- initially prescribe 4 hourly oramorph
- ensure breakthrough dose is prescribed ($1/6$ of total 24 hour dose)
- increase in 30-50% steps if patient is requiring extra doses or is still in pain
- convert to slow-release morphine preparation (e.g. MST, MXL) when opiate requirements established.
- if patient is unable to take oral medication consider converting to sub-cutaneous diamorphine - (3mgs oral morphine = 1mg diamorphine)

Anticipating side effects
- prescribe a laxative - softener and stimulant i.e. co-danthramer
- if nauseated prescribe a regular anti-emetic- (e.g. haloperidol 1.5 - 3mgs nocte)

Using Weak opiates for moderate pain
- ensure that a non paracetamol preparation is prescribed for breakthrough pain i.e. Dihydrocodeine or a small dose of oral morphine.
- as with stronger opiates a laxative must be prescribed - i.e. co-danthramer
- if regular extra doses are required go up a step to a stronger opiate

Notes:

1. **Pain unrelieved despite strong opioids**

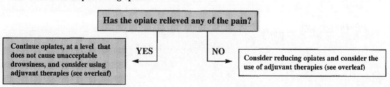

Has the opiate relieved any of the pain?

Continue opiates, at a level that does not cause unacceptable drowsiness, and consider using adjuvant therapies (see overleaf)

YES

NO

Consider reducing opiates and consider the use of adjuvant therapies (see overleaf)

*** Please see overleaf for further details on the use of adjuvant therapies and co-analgesics ***

. . . . /contd

Adjuvant therapies and co-analgesics for pain management

The choice of co-analgesic depends on the likely cause of the pain, making a detailed re-assessment of the patient's pain crucial. Below are some of the common pains that do not always respond totally to the use of opioids, and suggestions for their management.

CO-ANALGESIC DRUGS   **NON-DRUG METHODS**

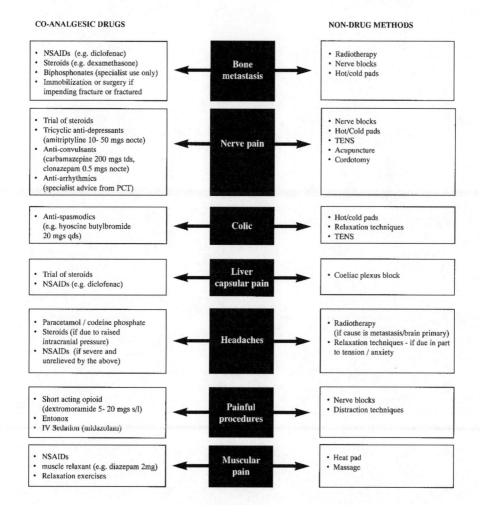

Co-analgesic drugs	Condition	Non-drug methods
• NSAIDs (e.g. diclofenac) • Steroids (e.g. dexamethasone) • Biphosphonates (specialist use only) • Immobilization or surgery if impending fracture or fractured	**Bone metastasis**	• Radiotherapy • Nerve blocks • Hot/cold pads
• Trial of steroids • Tricyclic anti-depressants (amitriptyline 10- 50 mgs nocte) • Anti-convulsants (carbamazepine 200 mgs tds, clonazepam 0.5 mgs nocte) • Anti-arrhythmics (specialist advice from PCT)	**Nerve pain**	• Nerve blocks • Hot/Cold pads • TENS • Acupuncture • Cordotomy
• Anti-spasmodics (e.g. hyoscine butylbromide 20 mgs qds)	**Colic**	• Hot/cold pads • Relaxation techniques • TENS
• Trial of steroids • NSAIDs (e.g. diclofenac)	**Liver capsular pain**	• Coeliac plexus block
• Paracetamol / codeine phosphate • Steroids (if due to raised intracranial pressure) • NSAIDs (if severe and unrelieved by the above)	**Headaches**	• Radiotherapy (if cause is metastasis/brain primary) • Relaxation techniques - if due in part to tension / anxiety
• Short acting opioid (dextromoramide 5- 20 mgs s/l) • Entonox • IV Sedation (midazolam)	**Painful procedures**	• Nerve blocks • Distraction techniques
• NSAIDs • muscle relaxant (e.g. diazepam 2mg) • Relaxation exercises	**Muscular pain**	• Heat pad • Massage

(Chemotherapy Services Committee and Palliative Care Team - November 1996)
WESTERN GENERAL HOSPITAL NHS TRUST, Edinburgh

Index